Inspired Thoughts
of Swami Rama

Inspired Thoughts
of Swami Rama

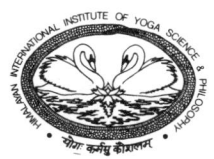

The Himalayan International Institute
of Yoga Science and Philosophy of the U.S.A.
Honesdale, Pennsylvania

Library of Congress Catalog Card Number: 83-080216
ISBN 0-89389-086-3

Copyright 1983 by The Himalayan International Institute of Yoga
Science and Philosophy of the U.S.A.
RD 1, Box 88
Honesdale, Pennsylvania 18431

Contents

Preface

This book is a collection of Swami Rama's lectures and articles that have been published in various periodicals and books during the past decade, when he was teaching in America. They have been compiled to make them easily available to the general reader who does not have access to the original sources, and to prevent them from being lost in the shufflings of time. All of Swamiji's significant published pieces (except his Gita and *Hi, America!* articles) that do not appear elsewhere in any of his English-language books have been included in this collection. The entries are arranged within their sections by theme rather than date.

"The Awakening of Kundalini" first appeared in *Kundalini, Evolution and Enlightenment,* edited by John White. "Energy of Consciousness in the Human Personality" was written for *Metaphors of Consciousness,* edited by Ron S. Valle and Rolf von Eckartsberg, ©1981 by Plenum Press, New York, and is reprinted with permission. All other entries are taken from Himalayan Institute publications and have been re-edited for this volume to improve readability.

Many people assisted in gathering this material and presenting it in book form. Thanks go to Barb Bova, Dr. Sudha Thornburg, Theresa O'Brien, Anne Craig, John Miller, and Linda Johnsen. Larry Clark copyedited the bulk of the text, and Patrice Hafford and Darlene Clark typeset the manuscript. Janet Zima designed the book, Dave Gorman took the text photographs, and the cover photo was taken by Dr. Ladd Koresch.

    Deepest gratitude is conveyed to Swami Rama for providing these profound teachings to American students and for presenting them in such a practical, understandable manner. The editor is grateful for being able to play some part in extending these teachings to a wider readership.

Arpita, Ph.D.

Swami Rama of the Himalayas

Swami Rama was born in 1925 to a learned and pious Brahmin family in a small town in the Indian state of Uttar Pradesh. Orphaned at an early age, he was brought up by a revered yogic sage of Bengal and was later initiated into his monastic order *Bharati*—"one who is the lover of knowledge." Trained to be a teacher, Swami Rama spent his youth journeying throughout the Himalayas, learning the yogic tradition and studying with masters of the major paths of yoga. He lived in the ashrams of Mahatma Gandhi, Sri Aurobindo, Rabindranath Tagore; exchanged ideas with Anandamayi Ma, Maharshi Raman, and Nim Karoli Baba; and sought out hidden sages to discuss the finer aspects of practice, philosophy, and attainment with them.

Swami Rama's formal education was also carefully pursued, and from 1939 to 1944 he taught the Upanishads and Buddhist scriptures in various schools and monasteries while studying philosophy and psychology at the universities in Varanasi and Prayag. He earned a medical degree from Darbhanga Medical School in 1945, and from 1946 to 1947 he studied Tibetan mysticism in Tibet. Having established a firm foundation in the basics of yoga, he developed intense interest in the science of *prana (prana vidya)* and the solar science *(surya vijnana)*, but his chosen path was *samaya*, a monistic school that is purely philosophical and that requires the direct guidance of an adept in *Sri Vidya*.

ix

Having acquired instruction in this science from his grandmaster in Tibet, he retired to the solitude of the deep forests of central India.

Officials who discovered his presence then requested him to accept the vacant post of Shankaracharya, the highest spiritual position in India. He agreed to serve, and in 1949 was installed as Shankaracharya of Karvirpitham in the South of India, a position he held until 1952, when he renounced it to return to the Himalayan caves to intensify his meditative practice. He spent three years of meditation in Cave Manali, journeyed to various holy sites, established an ashram in Rishikesh, and completed an intensive eleven-month *pranayama* and meditation practice while sealed in a six foot by four foot cave with only a single pinpoint of light shining in. With the inspiration and encouragement of his master, he then decided to bring the message of the yogic sages to the West.

Determining to unite his yogic knowledge with Western approaches, he traveled to Europe, and from 1965 to 1967 studied at Hamburg University, the University of Utrecht, and Oxford University, learning Western philosophy and psychology and teaching yoga and Eastern philosophy. At the University of Frankfurt, he conducted research on the anatomy of sleep and other phenomena, and he assisted in parapsychological research in Moscow for six months. He also served as a medical consultant in London, but his main endeavor began in Japan, where he established a major spiritual center that today has several hundred thousand participants.

Having completed this goal, he was free in 1969 to come to the United States, upon invitation by Dr. Elmer Green of the Menninger Foundation, to be a consultant in a research project designed to investigate the voluntary control of internal states. Hooked up to psychophysiological equipment, Swami Rama demonstrated his ability to perform feats previously considered impossible. These included stopping the flow of blood through his heart, radically changing the temperature of two points on the palm of his hand, producing various brain wave patterns at will, and remaining aware of external events during a state of deep sleep. His work influenced the establishment of new disciplines such as biofeedback therapy, behavioral medicine, stress management, and holistic health, as well as the new fields of transpersonal psychology and the psychology of consciousness.

The Western technological equipment and empirical paradigm were incapable of dealing with the more subtle practices and concepts that he wanted to share, however, so he decided to discontinue his work in this vein. Shortly thereafter he began lecturing in the Chicago area, and a small group of students gradually began to form. It was at this time, in 1971, that he established his own foundation, the Himalayan Institute of the United States. As the number of interested people increased, physicians, psychologists, and philosophers joined the staff and were trained in the yogic tradition. By 1975 there was enough support to open an Institute headquarters in Glenview, Illinois. The Institute rapidly expanded to include a dozen branch centers throughout the country and a larger headquarters in the Pocono Mountains of Pennsylvania, which hosts a variety of educational, research, and therapeutic programs.

Since the move to Pennsylvania in 1978, the Institute has expanded its Combined Therapy Program, its residential programs, its research facilities, its publications, and its offerings in weekly classes, weekend seminars, special training programs, and faculty lecture tours. In addition, it provides a master's degree program in Eastern Studies and Comparative Psychology in affiliation with the University of Scranton. Having established the Institute in America, Swamiji now devotes more of his time to writing at his small ashram in Nepal and to organizing new projects in India. A school where Indian culture will be preserved and taught is being established in New Delhi, study tours are being conducted to the Hansda ashram near Kathmandu, an Institute center is being organized in Kanpur, a branch ashram is being reopened in Rishikesh, a leper hospital is being planned for the Himalayan foothills, and there are trust funds and exchange programs being developed for students in India and America. His work to create a bridge between East and West thus continues. As Swamiji says, "We want to make people aware of the fact that life is a great joy, poem, and song, and that it should bloom like a flower for the sake of selfless service to humanity."

Lectures

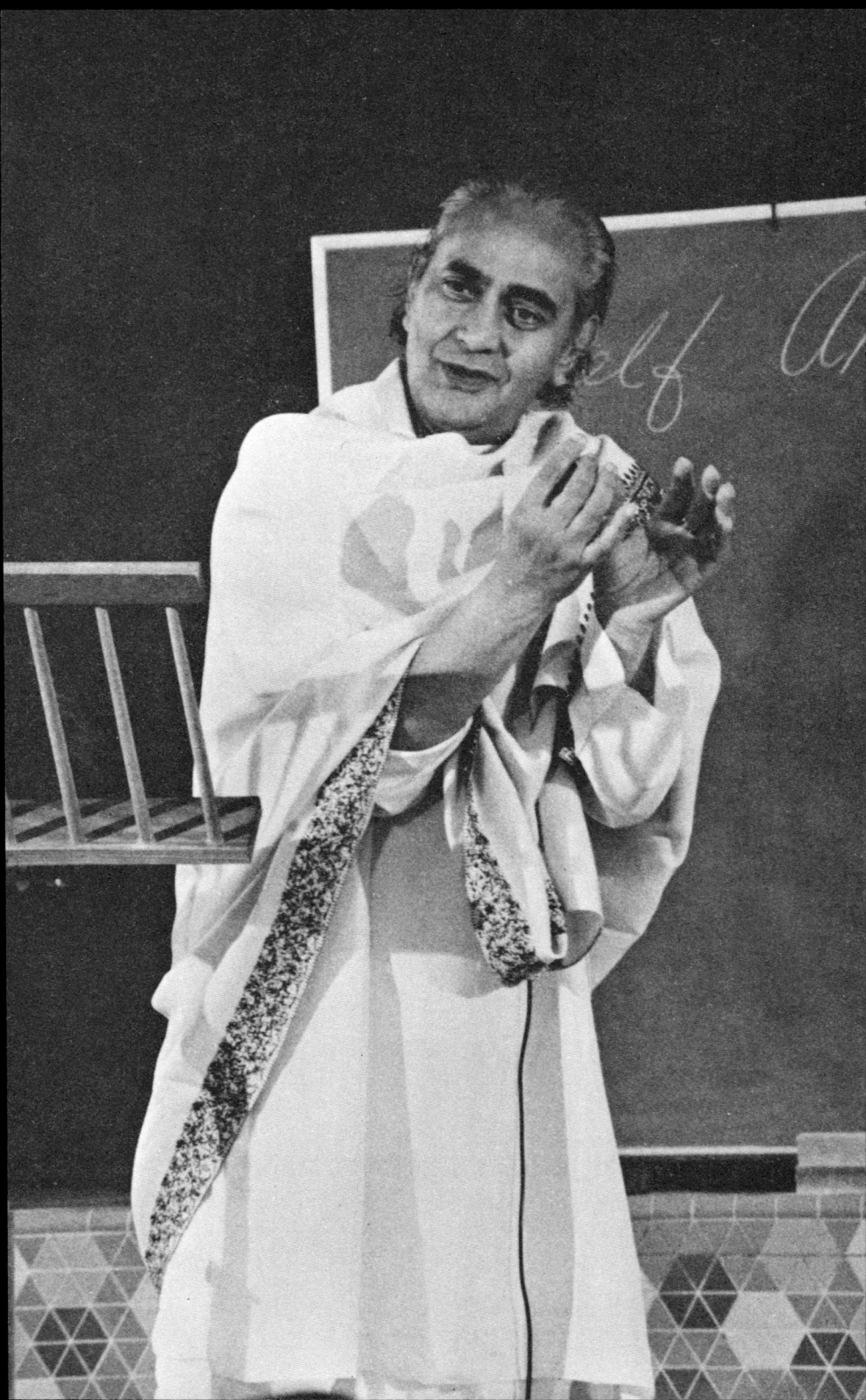

The Path of Raja Yoga

First International Congress, Chicago, Illinois, June 18, 1976

Yoga is an ancient word found not only in yoga manuals but even in the Vedas, the most ancient scriptures in the library of humankind. The ancient scriptures say, "The first being, the first manifested one, was a great yogi—one who knows about himself on all levels." Many people vulgarize the word *yoga*, but it is found in all the great religions of the world, including Christianity.

The term *Raja yoga* was first used by Swami Vivekananda, a great man who came to Chicago to attend the World Parliament of Religions in 1893. *Raja* means "royal," and this yoga is called Royal yoga because, unlike other systems of yoga, which are vague, this one is precise and systematic. Raja yoga was set forth by Patanjali in the Yoga Sutras around 200 B.C., and it describes eight rungs on the yoga ladder. Thus it is also called Ashtanga yoga because *ashtanga* means "eight limbs." In Raja yoga, philosophy, science, and practice are combined. Here it is the duty of the teacher to impart the principles of yoga and the techniques for practicing them, not by studying yoga aphorisms and manuals, but through self-discipline and specific practices that will help the student attain the goal of yoga. My master always said, "Do not teach any science without having experienced it. Then you will be able to warn your students. You will be able to guide them properly because you will be telling them not only what to do and the way to do it, but also that which should not be done." According to yoga there is no such thing as sin, but there are

3

obstacles that one must face. Raja yoga teaches you how to overcome these obstacles.

There are seven main streams of Indian philosophy, and the Raja yoga system is one of them. The first word of the first aphorism in all the systems of Indian philosophy is *atha*. *Atha* means "now," implying "now, then, and therefore." This word explains the whole truth of all the great philosophies of the world. It means that before you study Raja yoga or apply the science of Raja yoga, you should prepare yourself. But Western people have no time for preparation; they want to attain spirituality instantly, like instant tea or coffee. Many teachers therefore commit a serious mistake. They give students mantras and different techniques and practices, but they do not prepare them properly. Thus the students become confused and are not benefited. There are many varieties of yoga, and all are equally respected, but having many varieties can also confuse students. The truth is simple, but some teachers can make it so complicated that the poor students become bewildered. The Raja yoga system, however, is a scientific path, and along the path there are milestones so you can watch and see how far you have to go. It is a beautiful path.

The relationship between the student and the teacher or guide is extremely important on this path. If the teacher instructs you selflessly for your benefit, follow him. But if you do not find him selfless, and if he does not practice the ideals he preaches, do not follow him. A selfish teacher cannot communicate with his disciples truthfully. A true teacher is known by his selfless, loving behavior, for selflessness is the expression of true love. If this is missing in a spiritual relationship, then it is not true spirituality, and you should call it something different. A competent teacher is one who practices and who knows what he is teaching. See if your teacher is selfless. If he is, follow him. It is that simple.

Be an Insider

If you sit down quietly and calmly, you will come to know that the purpose of your life is Self-realization. To communicate with another person you have to open your eyes, open your lips, move your limbs, and express certain gestures, but to reach within you do not have to make any such effort. The easiest way is Self-realization, the easiest way is to "know thyself." But this is an inward journey, and for that, you have to learn to become an "insider"—one who fathoms all the levels of life and finally realizes the source of consciousness. It is so important to be an insider, that when someone comes to the monasteries of the Himalayas, we first try to determine whether this person is an insider or an outsider. We do not care how much he has studied the scriptures. We want to know, is he an insider or an outsider?

In the West, the educational system is very technical, but it leads toward the external world; it cannot lead inside. Man does not know himself, yet he wants to know the things outside himself. My master always said, "First, be an insider." Become conscious of this reality: your life is not external only. You should learn to understand yourself, your ways, your internal states, and your center of consciousness.

Patanjali, the codifier of Raja yoga, warns modern people that they must become aware of who they are. The foundation of the entire science of Raja yoga is explained in the first four *sutras* of the Yoga Sutras, in which Patanjali says, "You are identifying yourselves with the objects of the world, forgetting your essential nature." The moment you come to know your essential nature, you become fearless. Under the pressure of fear students ask, "Will I be enlightened? How long will it take for me to be enlightened? How long will it take for me to meditate?" They worry instead of meditating. This happens with everyone; it happened with me also. But my master told me one thing: "Be free from all fears." You are going through the procession of life. Why do you worry and bother for enlightenment? Start treading the path, and enlightenment dawns of itself. The first thing to achieve is freedom from all fears, and it is the duty of a teacher to give you that freedom. He should enlighten you with the knowledge of the true values of life, but it is your duty to prepare yourself for the teaching.

The basic concept of yoga psychology is to be aware of the

Reality all the time. Otherwise you forget your essential nature and identify yourself with the objects of the world. Slowly and gradually become aware that the Reality is omnipotent and omnipresent—it is within you also. You cannot cut Reality into pieces. That is the dualistic concept. Reality is within and without. There is only one Truth, and it is omnipresent and omniscient. Then where are you? You are in Truth, and Truth is within you. You simply have to become aware, and that awareness is strengthened by constant practice.

In the beginning there are practical problems. You start becoming more egotistical when you feel that the Lord is within you; you feel that you know everything and others do not know anything. You go here and there and say, "My master is great and other teachings are useless." These egotistical problems contract the personality, consciousness, and vision, but when you sit near your teacher and listen to him attentively, he resolves this problem.

Similarly, when you try to become an insider, when you start meditating and become aware of the Reality within, one of the first problems that arises is that you become an introvert, and when you become introverted you either come in contact with your suppressions and repressions, or you become egotistical. This is a practical problem that all aspirants face. When you become an introvert, you are not meditating. Not at all. You are just coming in touch with your superficial self, which is full of conflicts.

The science of Raja yoga teaches us not to identify with the objects of the world. We are used to seeing, examining, and verifying things in the external world, but no one teaches us how to see and look within. This is most unfortunate. According to Raja yoga, even if you start to look within, you will have to face practical problems. For instance, you may feel a lack of confidence. Fears and self-condemnation may arise, for whenever you close your eyes, you see yourself, you start talking to yourself.

My master taught me something very interesting that I will never forget. I would like to repeat it again and again so that you will remember, too. One day the ruler of a mountain state came with all his guards to see my master. It was about eight o'clock in the morning, and I was standing outside the cave. I was perhaps fifteen or sixteen years of age. I was brought up very freely by a yogi, and with a humble person I was very humble, but with an egotistical person I was very egotistical. To be frank, I did not have much knowledge. I used to imitate great yogis. The way they would sit, I also would sit, but I did not know what to do next.

This ruler came up to me and demanded, "Brahmachari, I want to see your master." I replied, "You cannot see my master." Get out of this place. Don't disturb us." The ruler's secretary and guards were shocked. They said, "Do you know to whom you are speaking?" "I don't care who he is," I said. Then the ruler came forward and very humbly said, "Sir, may I please see your master?" So I said, "You are most welcome," and took him inside.

My master remains seated the whole day, and twice a day he changes his posture. His daily nourishment consists only of a small amount of milk. When the ruler came in, my master opened his eyes and smiled, "Son, how are you?" Now, that man had been educated at Oxford, and he wanted to be like a Britisher and make polite chitchat. So he said to my master, "Sir, you seem to be very lonesome." My master replied, "Yes, because you have come." This reply shook him; it changed his whole outlook toward life.

When you jabber your whole life, let me tell you that you make yourself lonely. Your favorite people make you lonely. Those whom you love, and who claim to love you, make you lonely. This is a fact. But do you know that this is not love? It is attachment. Love and attachment are two different things. Love means giving selflessly, excluding none and including all. Attachment is possessing something. In reality, it is bondage. There is a vast difference between love and attachment. Western people say, "How can you live without attachment?" Well, you can live wonderfully without attachment. You can live on love. Love and attachment are poles apart. One is the cause of freedom; the other is the cause of bondage.

The Ten Commitments of Raja Yoga

In order to attain the highest state of consciousness, or *samadhi*, Patanjali describes eight rungs on the yoga ladder. The first two rungs are ten commitments—not commandments, but commitments. You do not have to be commanded to follow them by some teacher, yogi, sage, or scripture. You should be committed to them because you know what you are doing. So first, learn to know what you are doing; then start following. A blind follower will not arrive anywhere. On this path you come in touch with two sets of commitments: *yamas* and *niyamas*. One set helps your communication with others, the other improves your internal being.

Be truthful, be kind, be nice, be gentle—in my childhood I learned those lofty ideals by heart. But I did not know how to practice them, for they are merely words that we use to console ourselves and others. So my master said, "You should learn 'no'—that is, do not lie, do not do that which is not to be done, do not think that which is not helpful."

So first your teacher introduces you to the real teacher within you, which is called your own conscience. Then you start counseling within: "I should not do this because it is not helpful. This is creating an obstacle for me." The teacher inspires you, gives you strength—that strength which is already within you. The teacher introduces you to your own conscience and says, "My child, look within and be guided by this."

I can assure you, however, that the day you start counseling within, you will make mistakes. But so what? Life is not meant to be ruled by "don't." You have to make mistakes, and you have to learn from your mistakes. But they should not be repeated. Otherwise, confession has no meaning: "I confess. Please forgive me, my Lord"—and again I repeat my mistake and again I confess. This is not repentance. Great are they who learn from their own mistakes and don't repeat them. Not repeating is real repentance.

The yamas, the first rung of the ladder of Raja yoga, are: *ahimsa*—*a* means "no"; *himsa* means "killing, hurting, harming, or injuring"; *satya*—not lying, not doing things against one's own conscience; *asteya*—non-stealing, not having any thought colored by greed, which makes one selfish and egotistical; *brahma-charya*—celibacy of mind, action, and speech for monks and having control over sexual appetites for the householder; *apari-graha*—not expecting gifts and favors from others, as well as keeping the mind free from wanting to possess things that belong to others.

The niyamas are: *saucha*—cleanliness of both body and mind; *santosha*—being content with the fruits you receive from doing your duties; *tapas*—not allowing the senses to contact the objects of the world and thus create obstacles on the path of spirituality (senses dissipate the mind, and when the mind is dissipated you cannot attend to work properly); *svadhyaya*—study of the sayings of great sages, study of the scriptures as taught by Self-realized and competent teachers, and study of one's own internal states, actions, and speech; *Ishvara-pranidhana*—being aware of the Reality, witnessing the center of consciousness within, surrendering the individual soul before the universal soul, or expanding the individual consciousness into cosmic consciousness.

These ten commitments of yoga science prepare you to communicate with people outside and to be composed and tranquil within. Then you can start doing your work, start treading the path within—from gross, to subtle, to the subtlemost center of your being.

Asana and Pranayama

The third rung of the ladder of Raja yoga is *asana*, or posture. There are two sets of postures in yoga: physical postures and meditative postures. The student prepares for meditation with a posture that is straight, comfortable, and steady. The Bible explains it concisely in the passage, "Be still and know that I am God." I have visited many monasteries around the world, and some of them do not understand the meditational method, but in the Bible it is clearly written that the student should first learn to be still.

Pranayama, or control of the breath, is the next rung of the ladder. Once students begin to work with themselves, their awareness turns inward immediately, and they become aware of the breath. The study of breath is a very interesting subject. The Bhagavad Gita explains that there are two guards in the city of life, called inhalation and exhalation, that create a bridge between the body and the mind. As long as they function, one experiences life here, but when they cease functioning, that is called death. "Learned is one who understands the mystery of life here and hereafter."

When you start studying your breath—not only through practicing breathing exercises, but also through being aware of the whole concept of breath—you wonder, "Who is supplying this life breath to me?" There is only one center that supplies this life breath to you; there is only one proprietor of all these bodies. When a yogi becomes consciously aware of this fact, he does not hate anyone. His consciousness establishes itself in the Self of all, and this knowledge of equality flows uninterruptedly. He becomes aware of oneness with the cosmic center, who supplies breath to all. You cannot live without breath. You are freely receiving that life breath all the time. Actually, the subject of *prana* is different from and deeper than the science of breath. Here it is enough to say that there is a direct link between the individual and the cosmic Reality that supplies life breath to you. That's why the first thing that the Raja yoga and Zen Buddhist traditions teach their students is breath awareness.

Breathing is closely connected to the mind. You might ask "How is breathing connected to my thinking process?" I can easily tell you. If you suddenly tell me shocking news, for example, I will experience jerks in my breath. The motion of my lungs will be disturbed. My right vagus nerve, my autonomic nervous system, and my heart and brain will all be disturbed. The breath is a thermometer between the body and the mind that registers both physical and mental conditions. Once you become aware of your breathing process, you will find irregularities in it. But by practicing specific methods of breathing, or *pranayama*, you can gain conscious control over the unconscious activities of the autonomic nervous system and eliminate these irregularities. This is a science in itself, and it has a philosophy that is not learned through books. Only the yogis who practice it traditionally know this science deeply.

Pranayama is a complex subject, but even if you have only studied your breath, you will realize that you are not body and breath alone. You are more than that. You are a thinking being. In Sanskrit there is a word that you also find in English: *man*. It is called *manas* in Sanskrit, and it means "mind." The English word *man* is derived from the Sanskrit word *manas*. You are not merely a body; you are a thinking being as well. So your thinking process should be under your control. You should learn that all the modifications of the mind can be brought under conscious control, as Patanjali tells us. The last four rungs of the Raja yoga ladder are devoted to this end.

Control of the Mind

You can learn to control your mind very well, because it is yours—but do not try to control the minds of others and make them dependent. When one becomes dependent, one suffers, so you should learn to be independent, and you should not make others dependent upon you. When you have learned not to identify yourself with the objects of the world, and when you have perfect control over your mind and its modifications, then you realize your true Self, for control means to gather together the dissipated forces of the mind and to become creative and dynamic. Control does not mean suppression or repression. When Patanjali talks of the withdrawal of the senses, *pratyahara*, the fifth rung of the ladder, he does not mean that you should withdraw yourself from the world. Instead, you should make all your actions spiritual and change your attitudes and living patterns.

What happens when you have control over your mind and its modifications? Your personality is transformed, but you do not become abnormal. Patanjali is very direct and truthful about this. He says, "Then you will be established in your own essential nature." Once you have known your true nature—the center of consciousness within, from which consciousness flows in various degrees and on various levels—you are enlightened. To dispel the darkness of ignorance and attain freedom from all suffering is the philosophy of Raja yoga. You can do this when you have control of the mind and its modifications. Concentration, *dharana*, the sixth rung, teaches you how to control the mind.

When you start trying to gather yourself together, you will find yourself so dissipated that you don't have the faculty of decisiveness. This is why it is very foolish for teachers to say that concentration is not necessary. If you cannot concentrate, can you do anything efficiently? No. Your speech will be different from your thinking; you will walk in a different direction from where you want to go. If you cannot concentrate on a book, how can you read and understand properly? It is foolish to say that concentration is not necessary. That is escapism, persuasion, and exploitation. Concentration is a marvelous technique to be developed gradually and gently. It will make you dynamic in your daily life in the external world.

Patanjali explains various methods of concentration. When concentration strengthens spontaneously, it flows toward the object of meditation. When meditation—*dhyana*, the seventh rung—strengthens, it leads to *samadhi*, the ultimate rung to be achieved by the student of Raja yoga. There are various stages of samadhi, but after one has attained the first stage, he is no longer in the bondage of misery and pain.

Some students think that they can attain samadhi without practicing the preliminary steps of Raja yoga, but that is not true. No matter which mantra you have, if your technique is defective, if you do not have a philosophy of life behind it, then that technique can only make you a technologist, not a meditator. Work with yourself gently. As you look after your body, look after your mind. Proper meditation is very useful, and Raja yoga teaches that.

Learning to Unlearn

Once you start doing meditation, you will come to know that life consists of more than merely learning. You talk of learning— you say, "I want to learn, I want to learn." But that is not the proper attitude. There is something higher. On the spiritual path unlearning is much more important than so-called learning. What you really need to learn is unlearning, but only in meditation will you discover what this means.

I wish you could forget everything. If you could forget all that you have learned, in which language would you talk to yourself? What would be your state of mind? Do you know that when you have unlearned all the languages in which your mind thinks, you attain the state of samadhi?

With the help of meditation and through the unlearning process, you will come in touch with your unconscious. Gradual and systematic meditation will enable you to make your mind one-pointed and will give you the power to penetrate the infinite library of intuitive knowledge. Then you will attain the state of real joy and happiness. Joy is realized only by that mind that can fathom the deeper levels of peace. One who has attained such equilibrium of mind is never disturbed by worldly fetters because he has learned how to remain undisturbed, how to live here and now. He has learned to be here, yet above. If we live only here, we are flattened like a ball of clay and cannot get up, so we should learn to live here and yet remain above.

Do you know who is in samadhi? He who has no more questions. If you do not have any questions, if all your questions are solved, you are in samadhi, but as long as your mind is busy with dialogues, that is duality. If one part of your mind puts a question and another part answers it, you are not in samadhi. The day you are free from the argumentations of the mind, you are in samadhi. Samadhi is strengthened when you learn to practice your meditation constantly, without any interruption. This final rung of Raja yoga has led you to become the most practical of persons, for now you are fully free, in full awareness of Reality.

You are the architect of your spiritual life. You should learn to build it. Be brave. The brave alone enjoy the world. Learn to enjoy the world by living here and now. Atha, the first word of the first aphorism of Patanjali's Sutras, tells you to be here and now. Raja yoga says that you should learn to understand your whole being. You are a nucleus, and the universe is your expansion. You have to know the nucleus first, and then you'll know the expansion. The relationship of the individual with the universe will be easily understood after attaining samadhi, or union with the absolute Reality.

Self-Discipline

Yoga Sutras Seminar, Honesdale, Pennsylvania, May 26, 1979

The word "yoga" comes from the root *yug,* meaning "to unite"—to unite yourself with the cosmic Reality, with the cosmic Self. Because you are an individual and an individual is an unfinished being, you are incomplete. This does not mean that you are imperfect; it simply means that you are incomplete. The purpose of your life is to complete yourself, to attain that union which is called yoga. So yoga means "to unite," "to add," or "to unify." This word is not new to the Christian world, to the Western world. It is found, for instance, in the Bible as "yoke," which comes from the same root, *yug.* Here it means "yoking yourself to the highest Consciousness." The purpose of human life is to unite oneself with the highest Reality. Yoga is the systematic science for doing this.

There are two branches of science. One deals with the facts of the external world—how to verify and know things in the external world and come to certain conclusions. This is external science. The other deals with facts in the internal world. Yoga psychology, a system organized and codified two thousand years ago by Patanjali, deals with how to examine your own internal states. It answers such questions as, How do you think? What are the relationships between your body, breath, emotions, and thoughts? How do you see and perceive things in the external world? Why do you think the way you do? What is the nature of conflict in the human mind? What is the wall between you and reality? What is

15

reality? Does it exist? If it exists, is it self-existent, or does it exist because of another existence? These vital questions, which are not answered by any branch of material, external science, are answered by yoga psychology.

There is a great difference between modern psychology and ancient psychology. Modern psychology is only a child compared to yoga. There is no system to modern psychology; it is merely a collection of different and often conflicting theories, and it only scratches the surface. This is not the case with yoga psychology. Behind yoga lies a great philosophy, the most ancient philosophy of the world, called *Samkhya*. *Samkhya* is the very backbone of yoga psychology, which is four thousand years old and which has been repeatedly systematized and organized by many great sages.

Those who know both Western science and yoga say that yoga does not need Western science because it is already scientific, but Western science needs to understand yoga because yoga includes another aspect of human development, one that Western science does not touch. Modern psychology does not and cannot offer anything to the normal person—Freud, Jung, Adler and others all studied psychology to help the sick. But according to yoga psychology, even if you are a normal person, you are still incomplete. Yoga definitely has something to offer the sick, but it also goes well beyond the state of being merely normal and healthy. According to yoga, to be complete one should learn to understand oneself on all levels. One should be able to answer such questions as, Who am I? From where have I come? Why have I come? Where will I go? These four questions are not answered satisfactorily by any branch of science or philosophy except yoga psychology.

In order to begin to answer these questions, one should understand that there is a difference between the mind and the brain. They are not one and the same: the brain is matter, and the mind is energy; there is a vast difference between them. The brain is the seat of the mind, but the mind has another seat that can work without the brain. The mind is like a wheel that rotates on spokes, which are like the various functions of the mind. But the spokes rotate because of something that does not rotate—the hub.

The Faculties of Mind

In Western psychology the mind is described as a whole, but in yoga psychology the mind is described according to the various functions it performs. Therefore by observing the workings of your mind you can understand which faculty of your mind needs cultivating. For instance, there is one faculty that you come in touch with whenever you are involved with something and must decide, "Shall I do it or not?" That faculty of the mind that says, "Do this" or "Do that" is the decisive faculty, or intellect, called *buddhi* in yoga psychology. This is the judge within you. Its counterpart is *manas,* the indecisive faculty, which says, "What shall I do? What will happen if I do that?" Manas asks, "Shall I buy the book? Should I spend my money on it?" And buddhi says, "If I buy it, I will read it. I need it, so I will buy it." If you do not understand the coordination between manas and buddhi, you will always delay your decisions.

Thus in your normal life there are two people talking within you all the time. Sometimes your decisive faculty tells you, "Don't do this," but you have never disciplined yourself, so you do it. This does not mean that you are a bad person; it just shows lack of training. You do not realize that if buddhi tells you to do something but you do not pay attention, you will suffer for it. If your decisive faculty says, "Don't do this. What are you doing?" and you do not listen, your indecisive faculty will pull you apart. Which is stronger in you—the decisive or the indecisive faculty? You should find out.

Another faculty of the mind is *ahankara,* or ego. There are two levels of ego: higher and lower. The lower ego makes you always aware of physical, external things, and in this way you come to identify yourself with your body, you come to think you are your body. But is this body really yours? No. It has been given to you as an instrument by God, or nature, or whatever you care to call the source of material existence. The body is not yours. It is meant for you, and you should learn to use it. You should enjoy it. But it is not yours.

The fourth faculty of the mind is *chitta,* or consciousness. Most people are confused about this word—consciousness.

According to English grammar it is singular, not plural. There is only one consciousness, but it flows from its center in various degrees and grades, from consciousness of the ultimate Reality to consciousness of the physical body. You are an artist, painting continuously on a canvas called chitta—consciousness. Sometimes you are conscious of the Reality, and sometimes your lower ego distracts you from that awareness—sometimes your buddhi is not functioning; sometimes there is no coordination between the different faculties of the mind. This is because you have not properly trained and maintained your mental instruments.

Human beings have beautiful instruments to work with, but if they do not know how to use these instruments, they are of no use. You have allowed the instrumentation that you have to become rusty, so you do not know how to think, how to decide, how to understand what should be the basis of daily life. If your instruments were coordinated, you would understand that all the things you have do not belong to you, for they can be taken away at any time. And this eventually happens: everything is taken away from you—even your body. But for the time being these things are meant for you, so you should learn how to use and enjoy them. Then you will really enjoy life all the time. This is meditation in action. It is accomplished by understanding and coordinating the various faculties of the mind. Then you will be able to say, "All the things of the world, they are given to me; I should be grateful. They are given to me; I shall learn to use them. They are given to me; I should enjoy them. But they are not mine."

That coordination comes when you discipline yourself. Discipline means self-learning. You should be very sincere in learning and understanding. I am not talking about knowing; knowing is only a small part of learning. Learning means "to know, to experiment, to experience, and to come to certain conclusions and then be firm." Learning reduces conflict. Where does conflict come from? What is conflict? It comes when you cannot decide anything, when your buddhi cannot make decisions, when you do not know how the ego should be trained and used. Patanjali says that the various aspects of chitta, consciousness, the modifications of your mind, should be understood because they dissipate your energy and create unhappiness for you. He says that there is no disturbance in the soul, or spirit, which is always pure and calm. That which bothers you is in your mind. That which is to be understood is your mind.

Understanding the Mind

The first step is to be aware that you are constantly identifying yourself with the things of the world. For instance, if you say, "Oh, I am in pain, I am in pain," what are you doing? You are identifying yourself with pain. If you think, "I will die," you are identifying yourself with death. Why do you not see the other side? If you feel, "I will live," then you are identifying yourself with life. Your mind is in the habit of traveling in negative grooves. You are condemning yourself because you are identifying with the objects of the world, which are constantly changing, moving, dying, going toward destruction. If you do this, you will always be worrying.

It is better to understand that which is the immortal part of your being—the center of the wheel, the part of you that does not move—for when you know that this part of your being is not a myth, there is no more pain. And if you don't have any pain, any worries, any problems, what do you have? You have peace; you have happiness; you have bliss. But you are trying to search for peace, happiness, and bliss without first removing pains and miseries, and that is not possible. So you need to understand; you need to learn about yourself, you need to discipline yourself. You need to remove your pains and miseries—and then there you are. You have the instrumentation to remove them; you have the means. And you can do it. But you have to prepare yourself.

The first word in Patanjali's Yoga Sutras is *atha,* which means "now," "then," and "therefore." It means that, having prepared yourself, you are now ready to tread the path of yoga. So even before studying yoga psychology, even before understanding and practicing it, a student should prepare himself. He should be prepared to discipline himself. Many people, especially in the West, are afraid of the word discipline. They don't like the word.

But discipline means only that if you are looking at something, you should be fully attentive so that you perceive it properly. You should not be dissipated when you look at something. In human life, however, everyone's mind is clouded and dissipated because of the senses, which are outgoing. But the data supplied by the external world is not reliable, so people are in great confusion.

For instance, you see something but your friend sees it in a different way—and then you have conflict. You don't agree with him, and he doesn't agree with you, because you perceive the same thing in different ways. So you should be fully attentive. You should accept the idea that you will discipline yourself. You will not depend on the teacher, the society, the school, the college, the monastery, or the guru. "I will discipline myself"—that is the idea. Just have this idea, and if you go on strengthening it, the time will come when you can do anything you wish.

In the World, Yet Above

How can this idea be strengthened? According to the science of yoga, you should learn to understand the various functions of your mind. There is nothing wrong with your body, for it is matter, and there is nothing wrong with your individual soul, for it is spirit: the problem lies in the mind and its modifications. The mind is the wall that stands between you and the Reality, and to know your mind you have to know all its modifications—its various functions—and learn to control them. When you can do that you can attain *samadhi,* the highest state, and you can attain it in this lifetime. This does not mean that you have to renounce the world; that is not the point. If you have renounced and you do not know how to meditate, you can never attain samadhi. But if you are in the world and you know how to meditate and how to live a yogic life in the world, then you are exactly like a lotus—you live in the world and yet remain above, unaffected by the waters of the world.

But how does one do this? How does one live in the world and yet remain above? No matter which religious background you have, which philosophy you have, you must understand your mind and its modifications; and the science that helps you do this is called yoga psychology. What is wrong with human beings? Yoga psychology beautifully explains that all human beings are constantly identifying themselves with the objects of the world. You are constantly doing it—forgetting your true nature. And when you forget your true nature, then you suffer, because everything in the external world is subject to change, death, and decay. You identify with those objects that are not permanent, that are not everlasting. This is the cause of suffering. Anyone who suffers on any level suffers because of identification.

How do you identify yourself with the objects of the world? You begin by looking at something. You look at a tree; the sensation goes to your brain through your optic nerve and then through the brain to your nervous system and to different parts of your body. You get pain and pleasure. You identify with your body, forgetting your true nature. But all the objects of the world are constantly changing, and you are insecure because you identify yourself with those objects. For instance, you are afraid of death, although you never die. You do not know that you are immortal, that you are a child of eternity, that you are eternal. You have forgotten this truth because you are constantly identifying yourself with the objects of the world. Come home. Come back.

Human beings are all suffering. "This world is bad," they say. "The universe is bad. Creation is bad." But this is not true. Humankind has created misery for itself; humanity has created that whirlpool it is in and cannot come out of. The Yoga Sutras say, "Know thyself." You are fully equipped to do this, provided you accept that one thing called self-discipline. The Sutras also tell you how to discipline yourself; they do not impose discipline on you. There is nothing like a commandment in the entire yoga system. "If you don't do this, you will go to hell"—there is no such concept. All the great religions of the world tell you what to do and what not to do, but they don't tell you how to be. The yoga system tells you how to be. And the first thing that you should learn is to stop identifying yourself with the objects of the world. Stop doing that! Start witnessing yourself, and soon you will realize that you are different from your body. To do this you should learn to discipline yourself—to examine your consciousness, to examine your human power, human effort.

Discipline Means Full Attention

Don't impose discipline on yourself—"from tomorrow I will not lie, from tomorrow I will not take meat"—don't create such problems for yourself. Be gentle with yourself, because gentleness alone is strength. Learn to be gentle with others and learn to be gentle with yourself. Violent people are violent because they are not at peace with themselves. So be gentle to yourself. Then you will be able to express gentleness in your mind, action, and speech. It will come spontaneously. Discipline means, "I will use all of my instruments according to my capacity." It means, "I should learn to pay attention without any dissipation, distraction, and distortion. Anything I do, I will do with full attention."

You all like to enjoy what you do. Your whole life you plan to enjoy something, and you never do, and you have problems. Why? From lack of paying attention. Patanjali says you are constantly creating obstacles for yourself. When you see what happens because of your ignorance, you accept it as a sin—and then you give up. "I cannot do anything," you say, "how can God forgive me?" You have to learn to forgive yourself. According to Patanjali, you are not a sinner; so don't become weak. Do not accept the idea that you are a sinner; you are not. But you do definitely create obstacles for yourself. Be aware of this fact.

Patanjali tells us that we create obstacles because of ignorance. But what is knowledge and what is ignorance? He says that although we talk much about darkness, it does not actually exist; there is no darkness. Darkness means lack of light, but is this lack of light real? Go to the sun and ask if it has ever seen the darkness. The sun will say that there is no such thing. There is also no such thing as ignorance, for ignorance means lack of knowledge, lack of awareness. But if you are constantly aware, you are not ignorant. Constantly being aware of the Reality means knowledge of the Reality—and if you are constantly aware of the Reality you will never be afraid.

If you are afraid, then that means that you are constantly aware of that which is unreal. The word that you use most in your daily life is "I," and that "I" is identified with something called the body. So you constantly think, "I am a body, I am a body, I am a body." But Patanjali says, "No. If you identify yourself with that which is very weak, you are weak. Don't do that." Instead try to understand the Reality within you and be constantly aware of that Reality, and then move in the world anywhere you want. But that will happen only when you stop trying to find yourself within the objects of the world, only when you are constantly aware of the Reality within you. Can you do it in this lifetime? Patanjali makes it very easy, provided you have accepted, not the command, but the commitment to self-discipline. Pay attention to everything you do—full attention. Then you will enjoy life. When you are not paying attention, when you are doing something half-heartedly, you are not enjoying it. For example, you look forward to going on vacation to Miami or Colorado—but when you get there you think of your home and you think of enjoying coming back. You never enjoy being where you are. So don't postpone disciplining yourself. All enjoyments are dependent on one thing, and that is called discipline, self-discipline.

So Patanjali first makes you aware that you are constantly identifying yourself with the objects of the world, and that is why you are suffering. But when you start disciplining yourself, you begin to become aware of the Reality that is already within you. There is a state in which one is free from all miseries. This is the fourth state of consciousness, the highest state, beyond waking, dreaming, and sleeping. When you attain this blissful state, samadhi, you have freedom from all pains and miseries, and all your questions are resolved and answered. You are then free from all problems, for you are in a state of peace, happiness, and joy. Patanjali tells us that we can attain this state within this lifetime. But first comes self-discipline—learning to be fully attentive so that you perceive things properly.

Therapeutic Value of Meditation

Third International Congress, Chicago, Illinois, June 17, 1978

There are two philosophies in the world. One is called Western philosophy, and the other is called Eastern philosophy. Western philosophy goes toward the grossest aspects of reality, while Eastern philosophy goes from the gross to the subtlest aspect of our being. This is the only difference. Although we refer to Eastern philosophy and Western philosophy, we do not mean that Eastern people are different from Western people. People everywhere have the same emotions and share the same nature. The challenge is to understand that common nature completely.

To meet that challenge, no better tool can be used than meditation. Meditation is a process of knowing one's own being on all levels. From our childhood onward we are taught to examine and verify things in the external world, but nobody teaches us how to know ourselves, and we don't find any examples from which we could learn. Consequently, education today has become mere repetition and conformity. We continue to live under stress and strain because we do not know ourselves, yet we are trying to communicate with others. Thus our relationships in the world are not very successful because a very important aspect of life is being ignored.

A look at society shows that people who have attained many goals in the external world have not found peace within. For example, I once asked the wife of a well-known scientist, "What changes do you find in your husband since he has become

25

famous?" She replied, "He has become very egotistical because he thinks he has accomplished something." We need to understand why we have not attained a state of tranquility. It is because we have not learned how to be still. Meditation can teach us this. Many Christians say that there is no meditation in the Bible, but I learned Christianity from great Christian sages who said that ancient Christianity explains everything about meditation. The Bible says, "Be still and know that I am God." What a wonderful verse! If you learn to be still, you do not have to search for God because God himself, the godly power within you, will reveal itself to you.

Meditation helps in daily life also, because if we learn to be still we can release muscle tension, and muscle tension is one of today's major health problems. Muscle tension can create coronary heart problems and nervous breakdowns—not to speak of ulcers, dyspepsia, hypertension, and many other ailments. It is obvious that our current living patterns are very defective. And yet we blame others for our discomfort. A wife complains, "My husband is not behaving properly, and that's why I'm suffering." The husband insists, "My wife does not do her job, and that's why I'm suffering." Everyone is lonely. And we will remain lonely as long as we do not understand the reality of the *summum bonum* of life within us.

We should examine this fact of loneliness and try to find out within who makes us lonesome. If we search deep enough, we find that it is those who claim to love us and those whom we claim to love that make us lonely. Relationship is the cause of our loneliness; there is some defect in our relationships. And you cannot separate life and relationship—they are one and the same. Once we all understand this, there will be no more hospitals. We will be, though alone, all in one and never lonely. This awareness will develop within only when we understand ourselves on all levels.

The Levels of Self

When you begin to study yourself, the first thing you become aware of is your body. And when you become aware of the fact that you need a good healthy body, then you start looking after your dietary program and you learn to do certain exercises. You also need to understand that your body is constantly making toxins; those who know how to eliminate toxins are called yogis. Yogis understand the relationship between the body and the mind; they understand the relationship between the mind, the endocrine gland system, and the fluids in which the cells of the body float.

When you study this body/mind relationship, you will come to know that human beings are guided from within. You should simply become aware of this fact that you are being guided from within. You alone have the power to stand against biological laws and gravity. Your bones and ligaments, for example, allow you to stand in a way that fights the pull of gravity. When you continue to understand more about your body, then you can learn a comfortable and steady sitting posture. For three months, at least, you should practice sitting steadily and comfortably. Just learn to sit quietly and calmly. It is not necessary for you to twist your legs so that you end up having to go to the doctor on account of pulled muscles. If you can't sit in a comfortable cross-legged posture, you can use a chair. This is also a yoga posture, called *maitriyasana,* the friendship posture.

Sitting in a straight, steady, and comfortable postition will make you aware of your breath. Breath is a very important bridge between body and mind. Medical science is discovering that most diseases are psychosomatic. *Psycho* means "mind," and *soma* means "body"; it's the body/mind relationship that creates psychosomatic diseases. But what is between the body and the mind? Where is that book which explains the body/mind relationship? There is no such book. Our religious books do not explain how the body is related to the mind—no book in the world satisfactorily explains it. But when you become a student of life, directly studying life, examining this living manuscript whose beginning and end is missing, then you try to recollect and search for the missing pages of life. You try to study this living manuscript that is written by you. Then you come to know that the bridge between the body and the mind is the breath.

How are you breathing? What is this breath? This is a

wonderful science, but little has been researched so far on this subject by modern scientific researchers. Yet it is the breath that is responsible for the relationship of the body and mind. Two guards—inhalation and exhalation—are constantly guarding the city of life. Even when you sleep, these guards still remain awake; they are constantly working for you. When you start studying these guards, along with some anatomy, you will come to know that if you are not using proper diaphragmatic movement in breathing, then your heart is not being massaged or exercised properly. With simple diaphragmatic breathing you can constantly massage your heart, which is the pumping station to the storehouse of cells. More than ten million cells are present when you are born, but as you grow through life many cells die needlessly because you are not aware of this truth: defective breathing kills cells. The aging process can be arrested. You can live for one hundred fifty years if you understand the simple laws of life. After you learn diaphragmatic breathing, then you can progress to deep breathing and many other varieties of breathing exercises. Medical science has begun to realize the importance of breathing exercises. It now knows, for instance, that people who suffer from nervous breakdowns can be helped by being taught how to practice alternate nostril breathing.

After learning something about the breathing system, you can begin to understand how your conscious mind functions. Today a vast portion of the mind remains untrained, unknown, unexamined. We don't have any system to train that part of the mind that dreams. Our educational system is concerned with only a small part of the mind; it is not trying to train the totality of the mind. So only a small part of our minds are being educated and yet we call ourselves intellectuals—great, learned people. We have not begun to understand many, many levels of the mind.

The Journey Within

In the waking state we are not happy; in the dreaming state we are not happy; in the sleeping state we are not happy. Who is going to make us happy? We each pray to God, "O God, make me happy." But God says, "You fool, I have given you all that you need and you are praying to me! Learn to understand all the abilities that you have. I am within you and you think I am somewhere away in the clouds. If, as the Bible says, God is omnipresent, omniscient, and omnipotent, then where are you? Where do you live? Where is the place for you? You are in me and I am in you."

Be aware of this reality, that the great truth is within you. Then you are free from that dilemma called the mire of delusion, and you will be able to begin the journey within. This journey within—from gross, to subtle, then to the subtlest aspects of your being—is called meditation. It is not a religion. Religion teaches you what to do and what not to do, but meditation teaches you how to be. If any yogi makes meditation religious, that is his problem. People are always putting brands on everything: one yogi says, "This is my method"; a second says, "Here is my method"; a third has yet another brand—naturally the poor Westerners are confused. Meditation should be taught and learned scientifically and systematically. Then it will be very helpful for all psychosomatic diseases, and also for spiritual diseases.

There is such a thing as spiritual disease. If you study the lives of great sages, you will learn that even after renouncing everything, even then they had certain subtle fears—such as the fear of not attaining what they wanted to attain in this lifetime, the fear that there was still some fine boundary between them and Reality. So there are certain hang-ups that are spiritual hang-ups. Even if you renounce the world and say, "I don't need anything; I don't have to acquire or attain anything in the world," you can still have problems. Meditation alone can help you overcome these problems.

We are in search of rest and tranquility and happiness; but our sleep does not give us sufficient rest, and no joy of the world can give us perfect tranquility and happiness. Running around, confusing each other, we give false advice and poor suggestions. Today Easterners are coming to help the West, and Westerners are coming to help the East; the whole world has become a hospital, with the sick treating the sick. We have yet to find the solutions to the problems of humanity. How can human beings live here and yet remain above the world's limitations? How can human beings attain a state of tranquility and still conduct their duties in the external world? At present there is no educational system that solves these basic problems.

Let us offer a solution to this dilemma. Systematically start from body consciousness, and then once you understand how to sit still and perform harmonious breathing, you can easily deal with the conscious mind, that part of the mind that you use in your daily life during the waking state. When you learn to control that part of your mind, you are on the way to solving your problems and knowing yourself. At this point you cannot say, "How much dust is beneath this carpet of wakefulness?" You are only sweeping and cleaning the surface of the carpet. But when you progress in meditation, you will see how much dust has been collected under the carpet in your subconscious mind. You will come face to face with that part of your mind called the unconscious. The unconscious mind is vast, and only you alone can do the cleaning necessary to meet your real Self.

You will pass many milestones in your inner journey, and gradually you will come to realize that your teacher is already within you, and that is thy own conscience. There is only one teacher and only one life force. Don't confuse yourself by seeking out all kinds of teachers. The teacher is there within, and you must be aware of that teacher. Let your meditation introduce you to your teacher, and then that teacher will introduce you to God consciousness, to universal consciousness. Your journey through life becomes very successful when you discover the Reality within yourself, when you discover the kingdom of God within yourself. When you become aware of the truth that the Lord and Reality is within yourself, when you experience the Reality within yourself, then you understand that the Reality is everywhere.

Meditation Therapy

This process for realizing the truth has been explained in various ways by the great religions of the world, but meditation is not a religion. Meditation alone is the proper therapy for solving the basic problems of life. When psychologists realize that meditation is very useful, then it will be introduced all over the world, for meditation is perfect therapy. Currently, psychologists are using mere techniques of relaxation or suggestion. It is important that meditation not be confused with hypnosis. Methods of therapy based on suggestion or hypnosis were discarded by Jung, Freud, James, and other founders of Western psychology when they came in touch with certain forces that they could not understand. Hypnosis is not bad, but it is not a self-training program; it is based on someone else's suggestion. We are already hypnotized enough by culture. Our educational system urges us to learn many things, but can we forget what has been learned? Can we unlearn what has been learned? We know how to learn, but the method of unlearning is unknown to us. With the help of meditation, people can learn as well as unlearn; they can have perfect control over their memory. Then they can be considered to be perfectly educated.

When you have direct experience from meditation, confirmation from the outside is unnecessary. Then you won't need to ask somebody, "Who am I?" You won't need others to confirm your worth to feel secure. Meditation can bring you to the day when you know what happiness is. From that day you won't need anyone else's assurance that you are beautiful, for awareness grows with direct experience. Direct experience is the basis of a self-training program, and unless you involve yourself directly in such a program you will continue to suffer on account of many physical, mental, and spiritual problems. Drugs are not going to help you, because you are not body alone, you are a thinking and breathing being as well—and you are also the center of consciousness that is beyond these dimensions. A meditational program will help lead you to this source, from where consciousness flows on various degrees and grades.

Many people assume that meditation means not thinking. But if you stop your mind from thinking, you will hallucinate, and your mind will lose consciousness. Meditation does not mean losing touch with yourself or denying your thinking process. When you are fighting with your thinking process, you are not meditating. Fighting deepens negative thought patterns. Learn instead to let go of the thinking process; learn to gradually strengthen the witnessing faculty of your mind. In this way, you can understand and examine thought patterns with the help of introspection, strengthening those thoughts that are inspiring, helpful, and positive. Positive thinking creates a firm attitude for a healthy life.

Positivity is strengthened by someone who is already within you, whom you know but ignore most of the time. That someone is called cheerfulness. To have holistic health, you should learn to be cheerful all the time. Cheerfulness is the greatest physician. Do not fight; do not create negative thoughts. These two points should be understood and practiced by everyone. The dining table should not be a ring where people fight with each other. Anger changes the body chemistry and disturbs the digestion. This is very important. Learn to be cheerful all the time. We come to this platform for a very short time. If you calculate your daily life, too many hours are used in eating, sleeping, fussing with the body's appearance, gossiping, and going to the bathroom. Why should we waste our time like that? Is not human life meant for more?

If we can but understand the Reality that is within us, then we can eliminate worry and dissipation. Learn to be happy. Don't postpone your joys and happiness for next year, and don't leave it to God to make you happy. God is already within you; happiness is within you. Witness this presence all the time, and remain free from all fears. You are the architect of your life. Never forget that. By systematic practice, in three months' time you will be able to calm down your breath. Gradually, you will be able to have perfect serenity on your conscious level, and then you will find that infinite library called the unconscious mind slowly coming back to your conscious level. Then you can go beyond these levels to the very center of consciousness.

This is the process of meditation. The school of meditation is very helpful and essential for everyone as human beings. You should understand that the calmness, happiness, and quietness that you aspire to can be obtained with the simple systematic methods of meditation, which are very therapeutic. Everyone can benefit by meditating and learning how to be still—for stillness reveals the kingdom of God within you.

Mystery and Mastery of Mind

The Rotary Club of Delhi, Delhi, India, April 6, 1972

Modern scientists are trying to study the mind, but they are succeeding only in studying the brain. We have to clearly know the distinction between the two. The mind is energy, but the brain is matter; it is only a vehicle of that energy. A scientific study of the physical brain cannot tell us much about the nonphysical energy that is activating it.

There are many difficulties in the study of mind. One is that our educational system never teaches us to look at the mind as a whole. Even in modern psychology we are taught to take into account only the conscious mind. But the mind cannot be studied in fragments. The great Indian codifier of Yoga, Patanjali, has stated that the nature of the mind cannot be known by studying only the conscious mind; the mind has to be known in its entirety. Both the conscious and the subconscious aspects of the mind have to be known and mastered, and while it is comparatively easy to know the conscious mind, it is not so easy to know the subconscious. To know the subconscious mind we have to go deep within ourselves, and the process of doing so is called meditation. Passing through the waking, dreaming, and deep sleeping states of consciousness, we finally reach the state of pure consciousness, called *turiya*, the fourth state.

Unfortunately, there is much misunderstanding about the nature of meditation. There are no tricks that one has to learn for meditation. The process of meditation has to be very

35

systematically studied from both the scientific and the intuitive points of view. Such an attempt on a large scale can succeed only when the total study of the mind is made part of our educational system. Let us not think for a moment that this cannot be done. If the ancient seers could do it, then so can we. And it needs to be done. As long as true education about the mind is not given, there will always be conflict in society. If we do not understand ourselves we cannot understand others, and if we are confined only to our own minds, we cannot communicate with others.

Humankind has made tremendous progress in the field of natural science and technology. We have succeeded in going from the earth to the moon, and we may even go from one galaxy to another—but our longest journey is within ourselves, and we have yet to start it in earnest. To attain peace in ourselves and to make the earth a peaceful place to live in, we shall have to discover higher dimensions of the mind. This can be made possible only if we learn yogic techniques of rising above the mental level of existence. It is only at a higher level of consciousness that a synthesis between divergent and clashing entities is possible. There will be no peace inside or outside us unless we reach that level of consciousness.

Education in Meditation

There are two types of meditation: meditation in a quiet, remote place like a dark cave, and meditation right in the midst of our daily actions. Of these, the secluded type of meditation may be useful for the individual yogi, but it does not do much good for society. We must aim therefore at a meditation that we can practice while we are engaged in our daily chores and actions. We have to search for peace within ourselves and not outside us, and once we have gained this inner peace, no outside circumstances can ever disturb us, even when we are fully engaged in actions in the most difficult and complex situations.

All conflicts create mental unrest. A person who has not gained mental poise will suffer this unrest and consequently make others suffer also. Instruction in meditation should form an integral part of our educational system so that our children, when they grow up, can face the most difficult circumstances in their lives with equanimity and poise and lead a life totally devoid of tension. This instruction is necessary if we are to solve our national and international problems, because only a quiet mind can solve complex problems.

Learning Meditation

Our education today teaches us only to imitate. People are supposed to be able to do only what their elders could do. This hampers the full development of the young mind, whose possibilities are unlimited. These possibilities can be realized through meditation, which unfortunately is not taught in our defective educational system. Our educational system teaches us only to think, but it does not teach us how to go beyond thinking. As a result, we are caught up in an endless snare of thoughts that creates an ever-increasing tension in our minds. Our minds have been taught to work only in certain grooves, and so as a matter of habit they seek solutions to problems through more and more thinking, which results in greater and greater confusion and tension. As a remedy for this predicament, we have to give new and higher experiences and habits to the mind. To sit in meditation in a quiet place at a fixed time even for five or ten minutes every morning and evening can help one a great deal in learning the art of meditation.

There are different stages in the process of meditation. One should learn and master them gradually, preferably under the guidance of a competent teacher. First, one should learn to be completely relaxed in the body. Research has shown that muscular tension is the cause of ninety-five percent of all psychosomatic diseases. We search for the cure for these diseases outside, but the cause lies within us. Physical relaxation therefore should be the first step for better health of body and mind. Proper breathing is a great help in relaxation. One can be completely relaxed if one knows how to breathe correctly. Our exhalation, and consequently our inhalation, are generally very shallow, and as a result our lungs work to only a small part of their full capacity. Through the proper practice of breathing it is possible to acquire such proficiency that the flow of air through either nostril can be changed by thinking alone. Such practice will lead to a decrease in the rate of the heartbeat, resulting in a quieting of body and mind.

The second step in meditation is to learn to observe the train of thought that is incessantly rising in the brain. One should not fight these thoughts or try to suppress them, but should quietly observe them. It is a little difficult to do so in the beginning, but it becomes easier with constant practice. One should develop an attitude of complete detachment towards one's actions and thoughts. Only a completely detached person can have absolute peace of mind. Attainment of a detached state of being in which one is only an observer and not a doer will lead to complete relaxation of mind and body. Then one can learn to focus the mind one-pointedly. But concentration is not meditation, it is only a beginning stage of meditation. Concentration is on some object, but meditation is a state of objectless consciousness. While concentration usually leads to strain, meditation leads to relaxation.

In the third stage of meditation one learns the control of *prana*—the vital energy behind all our breathing and actions. There are certain special nerves and nerve centers in our body that, when aroused, give us complete control over our body. For this, one should learn the science of prana. It is only through meditation and yogic breathing that one gains control over one's inhalation and exhalation and thus becomes master of one's prana.

Through the practice of these stages, one gradually advances to the higher and higher reaches of consciousness, until one finally attains the state of *samadhi*—a state of pure consciousness in which one's individual soul becomes identified with the cosmic soul. In the state of samadhi one does not lose one's identity. In fact, as Patanjali has pointed out, it is only in the state of deepest meditation or samadhi that we realize our true identity. As a river, when merging in the ocean, does not lose itself but only expands itself enormously, so in a similar way through the practice of meditation do we attain a wider and wider state of consciousness, until finally we are identified with the cosmic consciousness. This is not a negative state of being but a positive state of pure bliss and pure consciousness. This state naturally takes a long time to attain, but it certainly is possible for those who aspire for it and who make constant efforts. Grace from above also comes in due time to help the seeker.

With a sincere desire and effort, it should not be difficult to learn the basic steps of meditation in five to six months. Future progress then depends on the intensity of aspiration and the constancy of endeavor. The result is worth the effort. If we are to have lasting peace, we have to learn the art of meditation.

The Relevance of Meditation to Modern Science

First International Congress, Chicago, Illinois, June 19, 1976

So often these days, spiritual teachers and religionists belittle science, but I don't agree with them. If you are a spiritual teacher and you do not have electricity for light fixtures in the building where you teach, I don't think anyone is going to come and listen to you. Nor can you travel from one place to another without a car, train, or airplane. Science has a place in our lives, and by condemning it we do not teach religion. The physical sciences are necessary for modern humanity, which cannot conduct its duties without the help of these sciences. Just as religious, philosophical, and mystical truths are important for the unfoldment of our inner life, so are scientific attainments a necessary means for our external life. Human life needs both.

These are two diverse sciences. One is called physical science, and the other is called the science of consciousness. The physical sciences discover the laws of the gross aspects of the universe, while the science of meditation discovers the internal states of human life. Human beings are citizens of two worlds: the world within and the world outside. We have to know the general laws of science to conduct our duties in the external world, and at the same time it is important for us to know the means of unfolding our inner being. The inner and external worlds are mingled; in fact, they are inseparable. Those who know the ways and methods of understanding their internal states reflect this inner wisdom through mind, action, and speech, and they conduct their duties efficiently in the external world.

41

When I lived in the caves of the Himalayas, there was confusion in my mind regarding the modern scientific way of living. I used to separate the scientific way of life from the religious way of thinking. But the day came when I realized that religious truths need scientific systemization, and science needs religious philosophy. All the great scriptures talk about the same truth, yet the followers of these scriptures remain unsatisfied and ignorant. Believing in the great scriptures and having faith in them does not give direct experience. Without direct experience, the study of the scriptures is not satisfying. I always tell my students, "You worry too much about enlightenment. Start treading the path of inner light."

When you tread the inner path you will not need a scientific instrument such as a telescope or microscope. Such instruments are of no use for seeing within. Seeing within is an entirely different art, and it needs no external instrument. Of course, it takes some time for one to become an insider, because our daily living teaches us to be outsiders all of the time. In our society today, success is measured by external achievements and material possessions. But if we do not possess peace of mind and contentment, all our other possessions are useless. We need to have inner tranquility and equilibrium to live peacefully in the world. I have met many rulers and rich men, but I did not find them in peace, and I did not find any happiness in their lives. Happiness is a symptom of inner peace, and peace comes through having a tranquil mind.

Meditation Techniques

All the meditational techniques described by different scriptures and taught by different masters are very brief techniques; by merely knowing the techniques, one cannot understand the entire philosophy that lies behind them. Meditation consists of a right technique, a sound philosophy, a strong desire to experience the Reality, and regular practice. The Desert Fathers as well as the sages of the Himalayas believed in meditation. The great Buddhist meditative tradition teaches meditation systematically, and the Christian Bible says, "Be still and know that I am God." There is no conflict with religion in the practice of meditation. The school of meditation is free from religious fanaticism, symbols, ideas, fancies, and fantasies. Anyone and everyone can meditate. Meditation is necessary for all human beings.

The technique that helps you in being still is called meditation, and the revelation therein is called God within. In India, children learn meditation by following their parents' example. An Indian woman meditates in her actions the whole day. Outside every village in India there is a well where the women go to fetch water. Each woman puts a vessel of water on her head, and on the way back from the well she may perform many different actions and activities, but the vessel does not fall down, because she remains conscious of it no matter what she does. If we also learn to do the things that we have to do while remaining always aware of our center—of the center of Reality within us— that is called meditation in action.

Meditation should be accepted as an essential science for individual and group therapy. It helps one to become a creative genius in the world and to have a tranquil mind all the time. Psychologists start and stop with relaxation, but the science of meditation goes deeper than that. When the deeper methods of relaxation are experienced, one comes to know that all methods of relaxation will gradually lead one to self-control. However, too much relaxation without conscious control can become harmful. If one allows one's muscles to remain relaxed for a long time, the muscles may lose their natural contraction. Moreover, relaxation based on suggestion is not a part of meditation; relaxation is necessary for meditation, but not the type of relaxation based on suggestion. During meditation, the muscle tone, nervous system, and various functions of the mind are brought to a state of balance and tranquility. The proper preparation for meditation is very important. That relaxation which gives you conscious control over tension and relaxation is the right method of relaxation. Meditation is an inward journey in which one explores one's internal states, finally reaching that center of consciousness from where consciousness flows on various degrees and grades. If the method is practiced regularly and systematically, it is not difficult.

Meditation Brings Inner Strength

All the scientific attainments in the external world, all the comforts of modern life, can benefit us if we view them as means and not as ends. Having the proper attitude is essential. Modern people suffer from self-created diseases, such as hypertension, ulcers, migraine headaches, and depression. The cause of these lies within the mind, and when the mind is trained through meditational practices, meditation becomes a useful therapy in daily life that prevents many diseases. When the mind and its modifications are controlled through meditation, one can enjoy inner serenity and do one's duties properly. Through meditation alone can one consciously come in touch with one's hidden potentials. To become creative and dynamic, meditation is very important. A meditator is never horrified by the problems of life; he or she is never tossed by the charms, temptations, and attractions of the world. A meditator remains unaffected in all circumstances of life, good or bad. Through meditation, every human being can do tremendous good for humanity.

The greatest obstacles in the path of meditation are created by the ego, and one who knows how to surrender the ego receives the higher knowledge. I once had an experience that illustrates the ego problem. There was a young man sitting beside me in a train. There was also a very old swami traveling in the same coach. The young man put a question to him: "Sir, have you controlled your anger?" "Yes," he said. "It's easy. I never lose my temper. I have no ego. I have perfect control over my emotions." But the young man persisted in asking the same question again and again. He went on asking, "Really? You have no anger and no ego? Have you really controlled your mind, action, and speech?" Finally the old swami lost his temper. He became very angry and shouted, "Shut up! And if you don't, I'm going to bang your head!"

Everyone's hidden personality comes up during odd situations. Actually, these can be periods of self-examination, and one can successfully handle such situations by being aware of the center of consciousness. To maintain this center consciously is meditation. Inner strength is higher than external strength. Those who have inner strength remain undisturbed all the time. The following story demonstrates this. I once was listening to a swami who was a realized being. He was speaking about meditation, and one of the students got up from the audience and said, "Sir, if I say that you are a fool, will you be disturbed?" The swami said, "No. I do not easily accept suggestions from others; I have learned to remain calm and comfortable."

A meditator understands gestures, emotions, thoughts, and desires. Such a person is aware at all times on all levels. Meditation helps one in facing the Reality. It leads one from duality to unity; meditation is unity in diversity. Meditation is sometimes confused with hypnosis, but actually there is a vast difference between the two. Hypnosis is based on suggestion, but in meditation we directly experience the Reality. As long as we see names and forms, we are under the influence of hypnosis. The whole of humanity is hypnotized by external conditions; we don't need more hypnosis. Hypnosis can help only on a superficial level. No method of hypnosis can enlighten a person. Hypnosis can put someone into deep sleep, but sleep cannot enlighten anyone. When a fool goes to sleep he wakes up still a fool—but when a fool goes into deep meditation he comes out as an enlightened being.

Students often ask, "How long will it take for me to learn to meditate?" My answer is, "How long will it take for you to light a dark room?" If you have light, you can dispel the darkness. And how long will it take for you to do that? A second. If you are fully prepared, if you learn not to waste your time but to utilize it for preparation, you can know the deeper levels of your being. All problems will be over if you willfully and consciously spare some time for meditation. A few minutes every day will help you in forming the habit. When the habit is strengthened, the mind starts flowing toward the grooves created by your habits. For those who have been doing meditation, the hour of meditation is the finest hour of the day. All human beings, in their ignorance, commit mistakes; meditation makes us aware of our mistakes and gives us freedom from guilt complexes. Meditational methods help us to become aware of both the good and bad qualities within us.

Another question students ask is about a guide or guru. Modern students have an image of the guru as a supernatural human being—an image that reflects their own ideas. A guru is one who thinks, speaks, and acts according to the dictates of his own conscience. The highest of all gurus in human form is he who practices and is experienced himself and who guides you selflessly on the path of enlightenment. The scriptures say, "Wake up from the deep sleep of ignorance, prepare yourself, learn to listen to your own conscience, and do not follow the tricks played by your mind." Do not waste time in knowing the different paths, but follow one path with all sincerity and faithfulness.

Inner Peace

Himalayan Institute Teachers Association, Honesdale, Pennsylvania, April, 1979

Inner peace and happiness is a subject that concerns everyone. It concerned the ancients, and it is our concern today as well—to understand how we can be happy. We always think that people somewhere else are happier than we are, but that is not true. Everyone is restless; everyone is unhappy. And the reason is that human beings have not understood the source of happiness. No matter where you live, no matter what you have in the external world, no matter how many things you own, if you do not have peace within, you will never be happy.

To understand this, you will have to understand two things. One is called "within" and the other is called "without." Accordingly, there are two concepts for living. One is: make yourself happy in the external world, and you will be happy within. The other is: make yourself happy within, and you will reflect that happiness outside. But there is also a middle path: you can do both. You can make yourself happy in the external world through your attitude as you perform your actions and speech in that world, and at the same time you can maintain happiness within by being constantly aware of the Reality that is beyond body, mind, and senses. Actual knowledge comes when you start understanding both.

We all expect to be peaceful; we all expect to have happiness within us; and that is why we like to enjoy things. Even the smallest enjoyment comes with the hope of finding peace within. But we

47

sometimes find that the enjoyments of the world create more turmoil than going without them would. Try to think of a single pleasure of the world that brings you lasting happiness, that brings you lasting enjoyment. You cannot. Suppose, for example, you have a watch. That gives you pleasure; but if you lose the watch, then that same watch becomes a source of pain. You depend too much on the things of the world. You think that after having this thing or that thing, after acquiring this thing or that thing, you will enjoy life and finally have peace. But it never happens. The things of the world cannot bring happiness; peace of mind does not depend on anything external, and without peace of mind you can never be happy.

So first of all let us try to see how our peace of mind is disturbed, how our mind remains in turmoil; for if we really want to understand our emotions, we can learn to be happy. There are many people in this world who enjoy life by being cheerful, by being in a state of tranquility. They maintain that state because they have learned to create a bridge between the external world and the internal world. People generally fall into one of three categories. Those in the first category do not understand the cause of their own turmoil. Those in the second category analyze the cause, but they cannot handle it, they cannot remove it. But there is a third category of people who know and understand the cause of turmoil, and who then remove it. These people remain free from inner and outer conflicts.

The Vedas, the most ancient scriptures, say that when our senses are not a source of distraction, when our mind is calm and quiet, when there is no inner turmoil and conflict, then we have attained the highest state of wisdom. Actually, the path of enlightenment is very short, but it is difficult to tread because we always expect that someone from outside will come and enlighten us. But this does not happen. Unless you are prepared to take responsibility for yourself, to understand your own inner being and your own internal states, you will not find happiness. You have to learn to do that.

Bridging the Two Worlds

Though the worlds within and without are different, they are not totally separate. So you will have to learn to create a bridge between them. If you do not know how to live in the external world you will never have happiness. You cannot, for life and relationships are one and the same. You cannot separate them. Somehow, somewhere, everyone is related to something, to someone. Even a swami is related to his practice. He has no worldly relationships, it is true, but he is concerned about his students, about their progress. We should learn to deal with these relationships. This is very important, for if we do not do that, then we are constantly blasting our inner peace. If we leave our duties, if we run away, we will still have problems because we carry our mind with us all the time no matter where we live, and the source of our problems is in our mind.

Some of you will say you have done your best in the external world, yet still you are unhappy. You should remember one thing: it is the ego that comes in the way of your relationships. For example, two people may have decided to live with each other, but most of the time they are on their own ego trips. "I want this," one says, and the other says, "I want that." That *I* and that *want* come between the two of them and create a problem. So in relationships ego stands as one of the biggest barriers. Modern egos are very strong because people do not get training in taming the ego. We all have different wants, and if we try to fulfill them without regard for others there will be conflict.

You should not expect to gain happiness from others. Everyone asks, "Do you love me?" But there is no need for doing that. You can find out within how much you love a person, and that is exactly how much that person loves you. Do not ask, "Do you love me?" That is not love, but expectation. You are expecting too much from others. Just love, and you do not have to ask the question. The whole world suffers because everybody says, "Do you love me? Do you love me?" You expect others to love you, and yet you do not love. Love does not mean expectation, love means awareness. If you are aware that in everybody's heart, deep within, there is eternity, you will love that. You will be able to say, "I love you not because of your body, senses, and mind. I love you because you are an eternal shining flame. We are like lamps, and your eternal flame is shining the same as the one in me. I love that flame." Saying "I love that flame" means that you are loving yourself when you love others. It becomes very easy. So you should learn to change your concepts, change your attitudes toward life a little bit and make it into a poem, a thing of beauty.

One of the sages I met in the Himalayas said to me, "I don't know why people are bothered so much; it is very easy to enjoy life." So I said, "What is the formula, sir?" And he said, "Life needs adjustment. Its goal is contentment, but those who do not know how to adjust—how can they attain their goal?" When you cannot adjust yourself in the external world, the whole problem lies with your inner understanding. So learn to study your inner processes, and then you will be happy.

But modern people have no time for insight. They do not want to sit calmly even for a few minutes. And if they do try, then they start thinking, and this leads to turmoil. But it is not our thinking process that creates the disturbance, that makes us petty and small. It is something called emotion. No matter how much wisdom you have, no matter how much you understand, it will not help you if you have not organized your emotional life. No amount of book learning can help you do this. Even if you know the scriptures, you cannot be happy if you have no control over your emotions. So you should learn to study where the emotions are coming from and why they are creating problems for you. You have to find the way to divert and channel these negative emotions.

One way to do this is to learn to control your attitude as you perform your actions and speech in the external world. Nobody knows how you think; people know you because of your actions and speech, and this is how you relate to the external world. So if you know how to direct your speech and actions, you can know how to live peacefully in the external world. The wound from a bullet can be cured, but the wound from a word is not that easy to heal. If someone is very harsh to you, or if someone has spoken something that you cannot forget, that wound is still there. Speech is very powerful; action is also very powerful. So only those who know how to conduct their actions and speech can be happy in the external world. Behind our actions is that which motivates us to perform them, and that force is called desire. If you are always saying, "I don't know why I did that, and I am sorry," then you are lying to yourself. You know why. Even if you do not consciously remember the reason for being compelled to do something, you still know it. Many of your actions are controlled by your unconscious mind, but any part of you that motivates you to do something is also yours, and you can learn to control it, too.

For Me but Not Mine

How do we perform actions in such a way that they do not become a source of problems for us and for others? If we learn to change our attitude, we will be happy. When we have to do something, we should find out how to do it in such a way that we are not attached to it. All the things of the world are meant for us to enjoy—but they are not ours. All of our pleasures and joys are marred when we start owning things, for if we try to possess things we become attached to them. Nothing belongs to us. That which gives us problems is our "my" business: "*My* house, *my* car, *my* bank, *my* this, *my* that." Wherever our *my* is attached, that gives us problems. We get attached to these things—and attachment brings misery—and then we cannot enjoy them.

Do you know that the words we use most the whole day, from morning to evening, are *I*, *my*, and *mine*? All the time we tell people, "I have done this; I am sad; I am happy; I am rich; I am poor. . . ." Whatever we do we always use that *I*. But suppose someone were to say, "Well, sir, you are talking of your *I* all the time. Can I know what that *I* is?" You would have to keep silent. If someone were to say, "Is that body your *I*?" you would say, "No, it is merely my body." So where is the *I* that you want to express all the time? What is that *I* of which you are talking all the time? Have you known that *I*? Where is that *I*? When you start studying yourself, you become aware that you have to know one thing: you have to know the *I* that is within you. And there is only one way of knowing it. You must ask yourself the question, "Who am I?" If you ask other people, "Who am I? What are we trying to do? What is God? What is Self? What is Self-realization?" they will think that you are crazy. But for knowing yourself and your *I*, you do not have to consult others. You have the power to find out for yourself.

If you put yourself in a completely dark chamber away from all light, then where are your hands? You cannot see your own palms, yet you know that they are there. What is that which tells you? Who tells you that your hands are there? Who tells you that you still exist? For knowing your own existence, you do not need any outside light. You have the capacity to find out within yourself. So first of all, you should learn to know yourself, and the ancients say there is a way to do this. If you were to ask a sage, "Who am I? Am I this body?" the sage would say, "No, you have a body, but you are not the body." "Then am I the senses?" "No, the senses are different from you." "Then am I the breath?" "No. Body, senses, and breath are not at all you." "Oh, then I think I must be the mind." "No, the mind goes through modifications—through the thinking process, through thought patterns, through analysis—it is constantly fluctuating. So you are not the mind." "Then who am I?" "You are seated behind body, senses, and mind. That which is peeping through the mind, senses, and body, *that* you are."

When you start understanding yourself, when you begin to cease to identify with your body, senses, and mind, then you will find that your own self is an eternal wave; your own self is a child of immortality. That which creates problems for you is your mind, because you are constantly identifying yourself with its thought patterns. You do not know, you do not think, that there can be something more, something deeper, higher, and stronger than the thinking process. You think, for example, "My husband said I am a bad woman. So, I must be a bad woman. My son also says I am bad. And my friend the other day told me I am bad. I am definitely bad." You have accepted these suggestions from outside. But you have not cared to make the effort to truly understand; you have not cared to look within. So you feel guilty, and you are suffering. This happens with everyone. You should sit down some time and think about it. Do not blame all these things on God, saying, "God made me like this, so I am like this." God made you beautiful, but you make yourself miserable. And you also have the power to make yourself happy. Both are of your own doing. You can transform your personality by understanding this.

Beyond Body, Senses, and Mind

How will you transform your personality? By being constantly aware of the Reality within, which is not body, senses, breath, or mind, but beyond that—that flame, that light, that life. Remind yourself: "I am not body, I am not senses, I am not mind—so who is there to create problems for me? This body, these senses, these thoughts have no power to create problems for me, so why am I suffering? I am suffering because of my association with the body, senses, and mind. It is all right to have them, to use them and enjoy them, but when I become attached to them and identify myself with them, I am bound to suffer." Suffering comes when you have something and you do not know how to use it. If you are aware of this, you will quickly come to realize that you have all the things you need; you simply need to learn how to use them. That is all.

So you should know the technique for using the instruments that you have. And that is, you should be constantly aware—inside—of the Reality. "I am beyond body, senses, and mind. Who is there to make me suffer?" If you say "God," then that poor God should suffer more than we because he would be responsible for having created a whole world of suffering. If you believe that God has created such a miserable world, then there is no need for believing in God. But God has not created a miserable world; it is we who have created a miserable world for ourselves. All the miserable conditions in the world have been created by us, and we can remove them and be happy. So constantly be aware of the Reality that is beyond body, senses, and mind. And when you do your actions, think that all the things of the world are meant to be used and should be used—they should be enjoyed. But know that they are not yours. Then you will be happy. Happiness is not something that we cannot have. It is our right; it is our birthright; we are working for that; we live for that; we hope to continue to live for that.

You talk of other worlds, other dimensions, unknown things. You should not do that. You should understand the nature of the known. You are not satisfied with the things of the world, but it is the nature of the world that nothing is permanent. Everything is subject to change; everything is decaying; everything is dying. Accept this fact—and then live in the world. Do not talk about the unknown. Do not expect the unknown to come and enlighten you; do not expect the unknown to suddenly drop in and make you happy. Make yourself happy by understanding that the light of lights is within you.

That which is called God or the Lord is omnipresent, omniscient, and omnipotent. If he is not within you, then he is not a great Lord, he is not omnipresent. If he is omniscient, then that means that the knowledge of God is within you. And if he is omnipotent, then the Lord in his full majesty must be within you. So that which you consider to be God is within you in his full majesty. You do not know that because you rely on your body, which is subject to change. But there is something that does not change—something beyond the body, senses, and mind. It is that light, that flame, that eternity—which is within you—that does not change. It is called God within you.

So remember, you are not so miserable as you have made yourself out to be. You are God, too, and cultivating this constant awareness within you will help keep you from false attachments, from identifying yourself with your body, mind, and senses. So you must say to yourself, "Body, mind, and senses are mine, but they are not me, for I am that eternal flame which is not subject to change, death, and decay." This awareness should always be with you.

So how do you live in the external world? How do you find inner peace and happiness? By creating a bridge between the internal and external worlds, by adjusting your attitude when you perform your actions and speech, and by being constantly aware of the Reality within.

Love Is the Lord of Life

Second International Congress, Chicago, Illinois, June 19, 1977

Those who are aware only of their birth and life on this platform of existence always remain afraid of so-called death. Yet it has been proclaimed by the great sages of all times and climes that death has no power to change anything except the body. There is only one power that can change the deeper aspects of one's being, and that is called the power of love. Love is the only center that radiates life and light, but we have not yet learned to understand what it is. If there is any universal religion, if there will be one religion in the future for humankind, it will be love, because love is the most ancient traveler of all.

When we examine the entire process of life, we can see that when a child is born, its first love is for its mother's bosom; then it feels love for dolls; perhaps later there is love for gaudy colors or certain styles. Then, as one matures, one develops love for honors and certificates from schools and universities, love for a particular man or woman, love for self-respect, and so on. We think that these loves are very necessary, but when we examine them we find that many times we are just feeding our individual egos. Finally when a couple in old age examine the whole process of life, they find that they have not known anything. They wonder, "What is next?" So love is that something which we feel and understand, but cannot explain.

The first commitment in yoga science and philosophy is called *ahimsa. A* means "no," *himsa* means "killing, injuring, hurting"; so ahimsa is an expression of love. Those who do not understand this commitment cannot love. If you feel that you love somebody but hurt him or disregard him, then certainly you are not loving him. To practice love, you have to practice ahimsa with your mind, action, and speech. We are often bewildered in our search for the definition of truth, and there could be millions of definitions of truth, but the great scriptures and sages say, "Why are you worried? Why do you not apply this great law in your daily life?" Ahimsa is so practical that we can easily apply it to cross this mire of delusion. We can go to the other side and enjoy that perennial center which is called love. By expressing non-killing, non-harming, and non-injuring, we are practicing ahimsa. Do it with your mind, action, and speech according to your capacity, and know that the highest of all powers is the power of love.

I have examined this for myself. Once, I meditated for ten hours and nothing happened. I prayed, still feeling I was different from the Lord. But then I completely surrendered and said, "Lord, I am Thine and Thou art mine. I am a drop and You are the ocean. There is no place for me anywhere." Then there came some courage from within, and that cloud of disappointment was dispelled.

Love and Fearlessness

I would like to share another experience that I had. In India, you'll find that there are many cobras in the jungles (though not in the cities, as you may have been told). I had gradually developed a phobia about these snakes. Whenever I sat down, I would look everywhere to see if there were any cobras; I even used to put my hands in my pockets to check there. How fear develops and becomes an obstacle to growth! I used to lecture on the Brahma Sutras, the highest of all philosophies, and my students always thought that their teacher was very fearless. But all the time my mind was going toward the groove of fear for cobras. I did not even speak to my master about it, and it developed in my heart for six years.

One day I said, "It is of no use to live like this, talking of the

highest philosophies and teaching meditation, but being controlled by the fear of cobras." And I started flowing tears. I was
outside our cave monastery in the Himalayas, and my master
came out and smiled at me. He said, "Look, tomorrow we have to
go somewhere." So, the next day I went with him into the
wilderness. After a while he stopped and said, "You have to
perform a ritual here." I thought to myself, "He does not believe in
rituals. What is he trying to do?" But I gathered some flowers
anyway, and he said, "You have to repeat a mantra ten thousand
times and offer these flowers." I asked him, "What is going to
happen?" He said, "First do it, and then you will see what
happens."

Early the next morning he said, "Pick up that heap of flowers
that we used yesterday." I went and picked up the flowers, and can
you believe that a snake was sitting on that heap? My Lord! My
whole body shivered. My master said, "Don't be afraid. This poor
creature has no power to hurt you. Why are you afraid? You are
hurting yourself by thinking like this, and your fear is attracting
him also. He might hurt you if you are afraid of him. Don't be
afraid. Bring him to me." So I was carrying that death in my arms,
and he said, "Look, catch hold of him." My God! I closed my eyes
and caught hold of the cobra, and he said, "Look at it. Have you
ever seen such a clean creature before? The cleanest creature in the
world is the snake. And it never bites except in self-defense. Kiss
it." I said, "Sir, I'm sorry, I don't have the power to do that. Can
you kiss it?" He replied, "Of course. Give it to me." I gave it to him,
and he said, "Look, now I want to tell you something. Sit down
here. When you are in deep sleep, why do your teeth not bite your
tongue? Why do your fingers not poke your eyeballs? Why do
your fists not hurt you?" I answered, "Perhaps our limbs are
constantly aware that they all belong to only one body." He said,
"That's right. And if you are aware that we all belong to only one
proprietor because we are all breathing the same vital force, there
can never be violence in the world. Anyone who is possessed by
violence will have to surrender before the person who understands
this."

Because I had been afraid of cobras, I had started hating them out of fear. Slowly, I started loving that snake. Now I know that there is a very fine distinction between hatred and love—a very fine distinction. This was a practical lesson for me that cannot be found in books. That's why I always say that a person's conscience is the finest of all mirrors and that direct experience is the highest of all teachers. Without understanding these two points, no matter how many scriptures you study or how many university degrees you acquire, nothing is going to happen; you'll not find any transformation.

Love Means Being Selfless

When we study the history of various great religions of the world, we come across an enlightened one called Buddha. In his time, there was a fierce tantric villain who was chopping off people's fingers. He wanted to use the fingers to perform a ceremony to attain special powers. When he had collected nine hundred ninety-nine fingers, he told his mother, "I need only one more, and I can't find anyone else, so get ready, tomorrow I need your finger!" The next morning his poor mother left home and ran away, and on the way she met Buddha. He said, "What's the problem with you? Why are you running with fear?" She told him the story and he said, "Come on. Let me go with you." So they went back and Buddha asked the woman's son, "Do you need a finger?" The son said, "Yes, and now I'll easily get yours. I won't have to kill my mother and take her finger." He lifted his sword, but he could not strike Buddha. Such is the power of compassion.

Though we all claim to love each other, a human being is very poor and weak as far as his claims are concerned. "I love you. O sweetheart, I could die for you. O sweetheart, you are a beautiful angel between the sun and moon." A man can compose a beautiful poem to seduce a beautiful girl, but upon examination you will find that such a person is selfish; he is using the word "love" for his own sake. Love is not selfish. Selfishness has built a boundary around us and made us captive. This problem is very serious; there is no remedy for the problem of selfishness. When we become selfish we start expecting something; a wife expects from her husband, and a husband expects from his wife. They call this love, but actually it is expectation, and expectation is the mother of all misery. Expectation mingled with attachment brings all the miseries of the world.

I have found that with all the great people of the world, though they have trodden various paths, there is a quality they all have in common, and that is selflessness. Christ was so selfless that when he was crucified he never said, "I beg your mercy; please release me." Moses, Buddha, and the other great sages of ancient and modern times have all been very selfless. When you are selfish you reinforce the boundaries that limit you and separate you from others. "I exist, I exist, I exist"—by this feedback you are strengthening the barriers around you, thinking you will thereby be protected. But that kind of protection chokes human life; it does not allow us to attain the next step of civilization.

The easiest principle to follow in life is the philosophy of non-violence and love. It's very simple. No matter how angry you are at the moment, later on you will come to know that while you were angry you were unreasonable and irrational. And this same truth applies to all people who destroy and hurt humanity. Love should not be understood as a selfish gesture. Love means being selfless, completely selfless. You can examine this. When you become very selfish, you will find your personality being con-tracted. Be completely selfless to cope with your fears, and you will find yourself in a state of tremendous power. So there are two laws, the law of contraction and the law of expansion. To become selfish is to follow the law of contraction, and to become selfless is to expand your consciousness. Constant awareness of that center called love is meditation in action. The highest of all therapies is the therapy of love.

Learning to Love

I always say that the institution of the family has been made by women only, but that they have forgotten their power. Unless women are awakened, unless they arise, humanity cannot help itself. The home is the first institute for learning, and that institute of learning is crumbling. So the first thing we should learn is to protect the institution of the family. It is where we get our first education; it is where we learn to understand. The child who receives love understands how to love. One who has never received love can never love no matter how many methods of acting he learns. Most psychological problems are sown in childhood, and the main defect lies in the education one receives. We should become aware of this, and we should ask mothers to protect this institution.

We should learn to respect motherhood. The finest of all symbols of love in the world is the mother. See the tremendous power that women have! If you put a stone on a man's stomach and say, "Carry it for a few days," he cannot do it. Yet a woman carries a child for many months. Then she is pleased to go through that death called labor. The center of her strength is the center of love. Physical pain has no value once you know the body is going toward change, death, and decay. The body doesn't matter to a real sage or swami. Even someone who understands this just a little can say, "Come on, I don't care about physical pain. I have many other higher problems to solve." If we are wasting too much time in eliminating physical pain, how can we get freedom from mental and spiritual pain? We have to learn to be strong, and true strength comes from within. We have corrupted our motherhood by cheapening it everywhere in the external world. That's why we do not get that love which no one else can give us—the love of our mother. We have to return to that institution called family life. If we really want to learn and grow and understand, we have to go back.

To be loved means to love. A husband may ask his wife, "Do you love me?" and his wife may reply, "Do you love me?" They may have lived together for forty years, yet they are still asking this question! In an Urdu poem it is said, "On the ladder of love, the first step is reverence toward the person you love." If you do not have reverence for the person you love, then you don't love enough. You cannot separate love from reverence. Most people have lost their love for life and for the center of consciousness.

Love Means Giving

Love means giving, giving, giving, where there is no thought of reward. To give wholeheartedly and willingly is called love. Those who have practiced this understand this law. Love means to renounce. It's like swimming. When you swim, you push water away from you and that is how you move forward. But what are we doing? We are trying to swim, but we are pulling the water toward us. This is not the way to swim; this is the way to drown. The principle of renunciation applies whenever we want to go anywhere. To get to that place we want to be, we have to leave where we are now. To progress, we have to learn to renounce. When we go on renouncing, we will attain that state which we long for.

Love actually means renunciation for the sake of others. The highest of all states is selfless love for others. After doing many, many experiments in life, finally one comes to know, "Why am I doing this thing for myself? It should be done for others. Let them be happy." And then enjoyment comes because others are happy. If you study the life of Ramakrishna Paramahansa, you will find that when he was suffering from throat cancer, Vivekananda and all his other disciples gathered together and said, "Sir, you are not eating and you are in pain." He smiled and said, "But you are eating. I'm very happy that you are enjoying." Similarly, when Christ was crucified, I think he was the happiest person in the world because he was crucified for the sake of humanity. When you have developed that sensitivity, then you cannot stop loving people and helping them. Great are those who help and serve others, for in serving others they express their love.

Once, when I was nineteen, an old swami suddenly came from the mountains to our cave as I was about to eat. There would be nothing to eat until the next day. We could not cook twice a day in the cave, and I had only a piece of bread and some vegetables. My master said, "This old swami is here; you have to give your food to him." I replied, "Look, I am not going to do that." He asked me, "Don't you have any feelings for him?" I said, "I'm hungry! I don't have any feelings for anyone." He stood and said, "I order you to give." When the swami started saying his meal prayer—"I am eating for the Lord"—suddenly my consciousness lifted upward, and later on I understood that in giving my meal to the swami I had really done something great. I started practicing such behavior again and again and again. Now, I assure you, if I am hungry and someone else is also hungry, I am pleased to offer my food to that person. We can practice this same thing in our daily lives. Let us become selfless and examine what happens during that time.

Love can be practiced fearlessly, faithfully, and honestly; and love alone can lead us to the highest state of consciousness. You are in eternal *samadhi* if you are selflessly doing your work. Fully do your work, live in the world, and yet remain above. When geographical boundaries have no meaning, when the world has become a small thing, when individuals interact every day in counsel with many others, which religion will we follow? I say that all the great religions are given by the same center of love. When we understand the essential points of all great religions, we will know that they are all one and the same. They all say be loving, be kind, be gentle, be truthful. Where is the difference? The difference lies in non-essentials. We can change the eggs, but the basket remains the same.

When we understand this truth, we will finally come back to the center of love and try to practice it. When we understand the highest of all yogas, we will know that it is called the yoga of self-surrender. Exactly as a drop meets the ocean, the individual meets the highest Being and expands his consciousness. We should look to that world religion and world government that will be guided by the love which is not merely animal or human, but which is divine. With such guidance, we will all love each other—including all and excluding none.

Emotions
and Their Positive Use

Third International Congress, Chicago, Illinois, June 18, 1978

So far, humanity has understood only three levels of being: energy, mind, and matter. Research has been done on these three levels, but little has been done on the level called the power of emotion. What is emotion? From where does emotion come? We are constantly receiving sensations from the objects of the world; those sensations are like pebbles thrown in the lake of our mind. Those pebbles, those sensations, are received by our optic nerve, then the brain, then the conscious mind, and finally they settle in the unconscious. They go to the bed of memory, and they settle down there at the bottom of the lake of mind. And when we want to recall them, we can. This process is going on all the time. That's how we memorize, how we remember. Our education does not tap those finer aspects of our being within us, so we have to learn to educate ourselves. Real education comes when we have finished with all these so-called educational systems—the basic systems that are essential for the external world but are not very important for the internal states.

Emotion is like a fish in the lake of mind, and when that fish is disturbed the entire lake is disturbed. When we become emotional we become unreasonable. This happens with everyone. We lose our temper when something repeatedly irritates us, and we become irrational. When we become emotional, our behavior becomes disorganized because the nervous system is affected. When we are angry, our nervous system starts shaking. And if we get angry again and again and again, many times in a day, we are hurting our nervous system. That is why psychologists today say "Let out your anger." But to let all that out in a disorganized way is not beneficial. How is our nervous system affected by an emotion that disturbs the mind? Why does it disturb our physiological coordination and then our body language? When we are angry, there is no coordination because we lose touch with our faculties of mind. What is that which disorganizes us? Emotion.

How can we make creative use of emotion? We have to understand that power which is called the power of emotion. In Sanskrit this power is called *bhava*. Bhava is life's essence. If we do not have bhava, we cannot live happily. We may be very good in our behavior, and we may also be able to perform impressive mental exercises, but without bhava we cannot enjoy life. Without the power of bhava we cannot understand how the flower of life blooms and how humanity also needs to bloom. If psychologists try to study this bhava on both sides, positive and negative, and start working in this area with their clients, it will be a great accomplishment.

So how can we study that? How can we know ourselves from within? It's not possible for us to understand ourselves from within without understanding our actions. Our emotions are reflected in our actions. "As you sow, so shall you reap"—this is the law of karma and actions, the law of all the great religions and scriptures of the world. Cause and effect are the twin laws of life, like two sides of the same coin; this fact cannot be denied. Though many philosophies try to cover this truth, it cannot be avoided. People can be known by their behavior, and therefore we can learn much by studying how a person of tranquility acts in the world. How does he or she live? How do such people sit? How do they walk? By studying our own actions we can also learn a great deal. By studying our behavior we can study our thoughts and then our emotions. An action is just like a thought; it is a reflection of a thought. Our entire personality can be analyzed and understood in a few minute's time if we use our common sense in studying our actions. How are our actions being controlled and who is controlling our actions? Our mind, our thinking process. What happens to our thinking process and knowledge and education when our emotion disturbs them? They become totally disorganized. So emotional power is a higher and deeper power. But what is the nature of emotion?

Desire: The Source of Emotions

The basic motivation of emotion is *kama,* the primal desire in man. Mahatma Gandhi, father of the Indian nation, was once asked by a writer, "Tell me in one sentence how I can attain the highest truth." He said, "Reduce your desires systematically, and go to the point of zero; then you will be free from all problems." Now, it is not possible to live on this plane of existence without any desires at all. So Gandhi advised, "Direct all your desires and resources toward truth, and you are liberated." To do this, we must first realize that desire can be either positive or negative, and we have to learn to discriminate between these. What is positive desire? "I am becoming aware that I have certain problems that are self-created, but I also have all the potentials within me to remedy the situation. I am the creator of my destiny, I am the architect of my destiny. I can overcome my problems. I am capable of doing it, I have the will to do it, I am determined to do it." These are sparks of positive desire.

Positive desire is creative and helpful, but negative desire is destructive. It is the source of negative moods and emotions. "I am good for nothing. Nobody loves me. I am lonely. I am dying very soon. What will happen to my children, family, and wealth?" This is the negative side. Negativity depresses us. And when we are depressed, our blood pressure goes down very low; our liver does not function properly; our right vagus nerve does not function properly; our heart does not function properly; our brain cannot function properly. If we are very actively negative, then we have hypertension. Don't think that your mind does not reflect on your breath and body. If you had EEG, EMG, and EKG electrodes attached to you and you were suddenly informed that your best friend had died, you would find that your breath would immediately become shallow, thereby creating irregularity in the motion of the lungs, which would in turn disturb the heart, the pumping station to the brain. The normal functioning of the right vagus nerve and of your entire digestive system would also be disturbed. This would happen with anybody. This is how mental disturbances and emotional upsets dramatically reflect themselves on the physical level.

Thus we are constantly hurting ourselves by accepting suggestions from the world. If someone says we look beautiful, then we are happy. When someone says, "Oh Swami, you are a great man!" if the swami is a fool, he will think, "Yes, I really am!" People are pampered with pride and become egotistical because of such suggestions. If the newspapers say that you are a great person, if people say that you are wonderful—don't believe them; believe in yourself. You can understand yourself from within, and if you really are a good human being and are on the path, if you do not hurt anybody and are progressing, then you are heading toward greatness. For there is only one who is great, and He is called Lord, Truth, or the Center of Consciousness. You are not great, you are only an instrument of this higher Self. The day you understand this, the world's suggestions will not affect you. You are accustomed to listening to these suggestions from the world, but this is not at all healthful. Such suggestions—"You look beautiful" "You look terrible" "You are a bad person" "You are a good person"—are creating a mask for you. One after another, we are wearing many masks, and together they make up our personality.

When we awaken and start understanding the values of life, with its currents and crosscurrents, then we can study ourselves and work with ourselves. When we start awakening, when we begin to be aware of the Reality, we start gaining knowledge. The greatest day of our life is the day we attain freedom from the suggestions of the world.

The Streams of Negative Emotion

The primary stream of emotion—*kama,* or desire—is the mother of all our problems, because desire is the source of all negative emotions. Desire gives birth to the stream of emotion called anger. For if a desire of ours is not fulfilled, what happens to us? We become very angry. Another stream of negative emotion is attachment. Attainment of that which we are attached to leads to pride, which arises when a desire of ours becomes fulfilled. We then look around and say to ourselves, "I have fulfilled my desire, but look at all the others around me who have not been able to fulfill theirs. I am someone great!" Thus pride comes to us when we gloat about having something others do not have. But when others have something we want and do not have, then the negative stream of jealousy arises. The next stream, greed, arises when we obtain a desired object but want more and more. Egoism is the next stream. It arises when we separate ourselves from the whole. Egoism is based on a delusion, on a false conception of reality. Actually, none of us has anything to be egotistical about. We cannot even create a small flower, or make a single blade of grass. Even our bodies are not ours. Our bodies are meant for us, and we can use them, but they are not ours. The proprietor of our bodies is that One who is supplying life energy to all. Everything that exists belongs to that One, and when we try to establish ownership over that which does not belong to us, we become egotistical and create misery for ourselves.

By understanding the source and nature of these streams of negative emotion, we can learn to steer our lives in a positive direction. Remember that intelligence has no power before bhava, the power of emotion. But intelligence, if properly handled, can channel emotional power so that we can use it positively. Learning to use bhava properly is essential to successful living. All the great achievements of the world have been attained by people during a particular state of ecstasy. We can do meditation for years and years and nothing happens; the so-called kundalini never awakens. But suddenly bhava comes and leads us to a state which is called *bhavatita,* "beyond." Then we fathom all the boundaries and go beyond, to the ultimate state of Christ consciousness, Moses consciousness, Buddha consciousness.

The Four Primitive Urges

If we want to learn to work with our emotions, we must first learn to quiet ourselves, to still the mind. We are not allowing our emotion to flow properly because the mind is continuously creating a wall, the greatest wall, between us and the Reality. We should learn to study all the functions of the mind and then study the positive use of our emotions. It's not difficult. From where do emotions come? They come from four sources: food, sex, sleep, and self-preservation. These are called the four primitive fountains. Now, we cannot say which is higher and which is lower. But each of us can observe which fountain has the most power, the most impact, in our daily life.

Why do we overeat? Because we are not supplying the proper diet to the body. The body is demanding, and we are not supplying, so we overeat. That is one reason. Or, if we are supplying a good diet but are not chewing properly, thinking that our liver has teeth, then we will not digest our food, no matter how good it is. Many of us eat the best food, but we never take the time to chew it properly, and so we take in larger quantities of food to satisfy the body's need for nutrients. If we learn to chew our food properly, we will not gain a "generosity" of fat—and if we already have it, we will lose it. Another reason people overeat is the law of compensation. Suppose our sexual desire is not fulfilled. What will we do? Quietly at night we will slip to the refrigerator, eat, and then go back to sleep. And in the morning we will swear we have not eaten anything. People overeat unconsciously. The habit is slowly strengthened, becomes unconscious, and then we give up, lose control, and say "I am helpless." So we should learn to eat a simple diet.

It is an interesting fact that food is given to the body first and then affects the mind, but sex is given to the mind first and then goes through the body afterward. Suppose a man who is very healthy goes to sleep and in his dream he has sex. If, upon waking in the morning, his wife should happen to ask him, "Do you want to make love?" he will say, "No, I have already had sex in my dream." But suppose this same man were to eat delicious food during a dream and then upon waking be asked, "Would you like breakfast?" He would say, "Yes, I am hungry." This difference shows that sex affects the mind first and then reflects on the body, whereas food is given to the body first and then reflects on the mind. The fountains of food and sex are entirely different.

If we are insecure in our life—if, for example, we are concerned about not getting enough food or if we are worried about what will happen to us next, or what will happen to us in three years—then we might try to compensate, we might try to find a substitute for our missing sense of security. We might, for example, become preoccupied with sex. No matter whom we were with or what we were doing, we would be thinking about sex. And if this thought were allowed to be strengthened in us, it could easily create disaster in our life. Now, I'm not telling you not to engage in sex; that's not the point. But I am talking about the necessity of studying how the basic urges operate in our lives.

Everybody wants to be joyous, but do you know which is the highest of all joys? You will probably say sex. But when people are tired of having sex, what do they do? Go to sleep. So sleep is the highest of all joys. Now, those people who work hard, who are conscientious in doing service to humanity and who do their duties skillfully, need to sleep very little. Mahatma Gandhi, for example, slept for two and a half hours a day. But when most people wake up they still feel somewhat tired because they have not gotten a perfect rest. There is something more that they are missing. We are not properly rested even if doctors put us into deep sleep by giving us sleeping pills or administering an anesthetic. No amount of ordinary sleep gives rest to the totality of our being. For this, we must learn to take conscious rest. We should learn to go to sleep voluntarily. That is called *yoga nidra.* Just as we can train ourselves in the areas of food, sex, and self-preservation, so we can train ourselves in the area of sleep. We can learn to go to sleep voluntarily and wake up at a predetermined time. If we build our will power by training the faculty of determination and say to ourselves, "I have to wake up at four o'clock in the morning," we will wake up at four o'clock.

Train yourself. Learn to train your will and let the will control all of your fountains. Then there won't be any question of "Don't do this" or "You have to do that." Whatever you do, you will do as a master. Today's world has enough food, enough air, enough time to sleep and enjoy things, but people have no capacity. They have no strength because they do not know how to regulate their emotional life by regulating the four fountains called food, sex, sleep, and self-preservation. If you want to be powerful and creative in the external world, you must learn to use emotional power for your enlightenment, to attain the goal of human life. You should learn to work on this; it is not very difficult.

Know Yourself

Now you understand how easily you can guide emotional power by having a little bit of knowledge about food, by regulating your sleep and your sex life, and by understanding your needs, your body, and your mind. I am not telling you to go to a monastery. When I go to monasteries, I find the monks talking about the world. They say, "Hey, have you seen New York? What is it like there?" I reply, "Why are you concerned? Here you are in a monastery, and yet you are talking about the world!" Then when I go to New York I find people there talking about monasteries. Nobody has peace. For peace you need not run away, leave your home, sit under the tree, go visit a monastery, or live in the Himalayas. That is all false and untrue. Instead, you should learn to organize your actions, thinking process, and emotions, and learn to be creative wherever you are.

Never forget these words: this body is a shrine and He who dwells within, the light within, is the bright Being in you. Know Him first. The day you are eager to know, the day you are anxious to know, the day you commit yourself to making Self-realization the goal of your life, what will you become? Will you change your religion? No. It doesn't need to be changed. Whether you are Christian, Hindu, Buddhist, or Jew, the goal is the same: "Know thyself." By knowing yourself, you know the Self of all. Then you can truly communicate with others.

We are not communicating with each other because we do not know ourselves, and thus we do not know how to present ourselves properly or understand others properly. This is a great problem. We are constantly talking about love, but without understanding ourselves we cannot give love to others or recieve love from them. We are lonely because we do not know ourselves. We want friends to make us happy, but nobody can make anybody else happy. Happiness is your own creation, and you are the creation of the Lord. Never forget that.

There are positive powers within you; the power of emotion is a wonderful power. If you learn how to use it positively, it can enlighten you in a second's time. Buddha said, "Learn to light thy own lamp. No one else can give you salvation." You have simply to know the light that burns in this lamp of life. Direct your emotions upward toward awareness. Ask yourself, "Am I only a body? No. Then who am I? I have a body, senses, and a mind, but I am not them. Then who am I? I am that light, the light of life—that perennial light, that everlasting light which is not subject to change, death, and decay." When we become free from all fears, then we understand the purpose of life. Then we have the capacity to organize our emotions by understanding, by regulating our four main appetites. It's a simple thing.

Not all saints have been renunciates or clergymen. Some have been able to live as saints in the world because they knew how to organize, control, and direct their appetites. Anybody who can do that is free here and now. Such a person remains above like a lotus, the symbol of yoga science. The lotus grows in the mud and the water but keeps its petals free from the effect of the water and the mud. We human beings have that capacity, but it will not be realized as long as we limit ourselves to matter, energy, and mind. We have yet to learn to understand bhava, the power of emotion. The way to do this has been explained beautifully by a sage in Punjab whose name was Bollesha. Someone once asked him, "Sir, tell me, how can I attain God?" He said, "Why are you bewildered? It is very easy to attain the Reality: simply disconnect yourself here [pointing down] and connect yourself there [pointing up]."

Only your attitudes toward life, toward the world, need to be changed; you have not to change yourself. Nothing should be changed. You are you, your mother is your mother, your father is your father, your children are your children, your friends are your friends. There is no need for any of them to be changed. Only your attitudes toward them should be changed. Learn to change your attitude toward the world. Be wherever you are, but learn to understand one principle of life: "All the things of the world are meant for me. I should learn to use them, but I should not be attached." For instance, I am now using this auditorium. Is it mine? No. But I have the right to use it. Learn to enjoy life by understanding this principle. Live in the world, love all the things of the world, but realize that they are not yours, and do not be attached to them. This philosophy of life is very simple; we should learn to apply it. The world is a beautiful thing. That's why it distracts you. A powerful person learns how to live in it yet remain above. A true master is one who knows how to live in the world yet remain out of it.

The Finest Emotion Is Love

It's easy to control and direct emotions for creative use provided we have channeled the negative emotions properly and allowed the positive emotions to flow. Then we can learn to give, learn to love. Self-surrender is the highest of all yogas. As long as we have not surrendered our mere self to the highest Self, we cannot learn anything. Just surrender yourself. There are three steps of realization. The first is "Please accept me, Lord. I am Thine." Then, when we become more sure of the Reality, the concept becomes "Thou art mine, Thou art mine, Thou art mine." And after we have attained this state, the final stage is "I and my Father are one"; *Tat tvam asi:* "That thou art." When Christ said, "I and my Father are one," he was in that state of oneness. And when he said, "This is not my power, this is the power of my Father; that is how I am able to heal you," he was in the state of "Thou art mine." These stages are not to be merely spoken about: they are to be realized.

Studying the lives of great sages can be helpful when we are practicing in our own lives, when we ourselves are treading the path of light. Such study shows us that *bhava bhakti,* love, is essential for all paths. Love is the key to leading a joyous, meaningful, and creative life. What is love? The finest emotion is love. The positive part of emotion is love. In a worldly sense, it is an itching of the heart that can never be scratched. Fingers cannot reach there. It is inexplicable. You cannot express it, for the avenues of expression are limited. They cannot express that warmth which you feel within. But that love should not be mingled with selfishness. If you are wanting something, you are not loving. Loving means giving, giving, giving, giving. Love does not believe in taking, but just giving. When we completely give, we have given up everything and we give everything. That is called love.

But what do we do in our daily life? A wife expects her husband to love her, and her husband expects to be loved. But you know, that's not love; that's expectation. Expectation is the mother of all miseries, but love is the mother of freedom. Learn to love without expectation. Or if you cannot live without it, expect little and love more. Don't expect too much reward from love; the reward for love comes after death, not in one's lifetime. A lover is one who silently gives all that he or she has. Such people don't talk about the next world, for they are liberated here and now. When you learn to direct your emotions, when you learn the positive power of emotion, when you learn to love, then you will remember one thing: surrender everything that you have. Anything that you think is yours, surrender it, saying, "It is Thine, Thine, Thine." The easiest path is the path of self-surrender. The dawn of Christ consciousness comes when you surrender yourself and empty yourself and allow the Reality to come in.

Do you know what a flute is like? If we put a small plug in a flute it will not play. You say, "I have so many weaknesses." Don't worry. You are like a flute having many holes; it will play if you don't allow anything to remain inside. That's all. You'll never find a human being who is perfect. A human being is an unfinished being, an unfinished creature. You should learn to surrender. Don't condemn yourself by saying, "I don't know anything; I don't have wisdom; I am ignorant; I am guilty; I am weak," and so on. Don't suffer like that—you have no right to do that. Just surrender by accepting the higher Reality in daily life, and enjoy. This is called *sadhana*—spiritual practice—in the world here and now.

Positive use of emotion means directing our love, directing our emotion, toward creative use by becoming a real lover, a lover of humanity. What is the sign of such a lover? A lover of humanity is that person who has given everything to humanity. And if you once acquire that taste, I tell you, you cannot live without it ever again. Then no matter how many times the world persecutes you, that persecution is a joy, pain is a joy, and you live happily, for you have gone beyond these relative terms. There comes a time when what you today call pain is no longer experienced as pain. There is no pain after you attain the state of joy. What is pain? What is death? Suppose someone wants to kill me—they cannot. They can take away my body—it's no more to me than my garment. But how can anyone kill me? How can anyone kill the immortal? Challenge death and say, "O Mother, you have no power to torture me. Accept me in your lap; put me into deep *samadhi.*" So death becomes a part of samadhi; there is no pain for you.

Learn to understand. Try to be a great lover of humanity. The sign and symptom of such a person is selflessness. The one characteristic that all great people of the world have in common is complete selflessness. Such people do everything for the sake of others. They live to love others. That is called liberation here and now. By understanding, analyzing, and directing the emotional power, it is possible for each of us to become creative and successful in the world and to attain the highest state within.

Desirelessness

Himalayan Institute, Glenview, Illinois, July 19, 1974

The most important thing in life is to achieve perennial peace within. Life is not fulfilled until we are able to remain in constant peace, and that peace can be found within us even in the midst of activity. But most of us are lost in the pursuit of worldly goals and do not remember this. So often our energies, resources, potentials are wasted because we do not remain aware of our central purpose. We are constantly identifying ourselves with the objects of the world and forgetting our real Self within. To attain peace it is not necessary that we obtain anything new—we simply need to cease identifying ourselves with that which is not ours.

To have this peace is to attain the state called desirelessness. Desire is the source of motivation in our lives, so dealing directly with desire is most important. Normally we only make efforts to fulfill our desires, and we do not try to understand their real nature; but peace of mind is possible only when we give up fulfilling these desires for some time. When we sit down and examine within ourselves, we see that there are really very few desires. Learning to deal with these desires, and strengthening that desire which is actually the prime desire in life, leads us to fulfill the purpose of life and to attain the highest state of wisdom, peace, and bliss, the state that is free from all pains and bondage.

The purpose of practicing meditation is to attain that height where there are no desires. As long as we have desires, we cannot attain the deeper and higher levels of life. I have never seen peace in anyone as long as their desires remain in the active state. Meditation leads to peace, happiness, and bliss. It leads to freedom from all pains and direct experience of the highest knowledge. But all that comes only after we obtain the height called desirelessness. Actual meditation starts only when we have attained a state of desirelessness, and anything before this is only a step on the way to meditation.

Once I became very dissatisfied with the results of my meditation and desperately desired to see God. So I approached my master and said, "If you are really someone great, you should show me God. Why should I follow you if you do not show me God?" So he answered, "I promise to show you God tomorrow morning." I had always been very punctual in my practices, my ablutions, and my meditation, but after this talk with my master I said, "What is the use of meditating now? Tomorrow morning I am seeing God." And I could not sleep in that excitement. In the morning my master asked, "How did you pass the night?" I answered, "Very restlessly." He said, "That is not a sign of being ready to see God! If you are so excited by your desire to see God that you cannot sleep, you don't have peace of mind. How can you see God if you don't have a peaceful mind?" I asked him, "Are you still going to show me God?" "Yes," he responded, "I promised you I would. Can you tell me what kind of God you want to see?" I could not explain to my master what kind of God I wanted to see, even though there are volumes of scriptures that talk about God. Some say He is abstract; some say He is particular or personal; some say He is all that is. Finally I recited a verse from the ancient scriptures that said, "Full of peace, full of happiness, and full of bliss." Then he said to me, "But that is within you! And you are searching for it somewhere outside yourself in mundane life. You are searching for God in the wrong place!" So you see, in that way our desires—even our desire to know God—keep us from attaining the highest wisdom that is within ourselves.

Love and Nonattachment

Because we do not understand and control our desires, we do not know what love is. Love is not possible without nonattachment, which is little understood or practiced. Love dawns when nonattachment becomes strengthened. All the belongings of the world may then remain with us as they are, but our way of relating to them changes because we understand their proper use and value. We should learn to do our duties skillfully and selflessly by understanding that all the things of the world are meant for our use and that we should learn to use these things as means to attain the highest end. We should not establish proprietorship over the things that we have. Attachment to the things of the world stands in the way of our highest development. We actually do not need any of these external things for our growth and enlightenment. They are for our use, not our ownership.

We have simply to be always aware of the Truth, for awareness of Truth is real knowledge, and lack of awareness is ignorance. All of the anxieties, agonies, and problems that you experience are there because you are not constantly aware of the Reality that is within us all the time. Do you understand the nature of your search? If you do not understand the nature of that center for which you are searching, your whole life can be spent in searching without ever attaining God. Do not delay in realizing the happiness within. To be aware of the here and now, and thereby find peace, is the purpose of life. You can attain it. But we have not formed the habit of living in the now; we are constantly brooding on the past or imagining about the future. Try to live here and now. Every moment is joyous, every moment is wonderful! Every moment is full of life—so let the flower of life bloom. If you can remain here and now, that is called meditation. In meditation there is no time at all; there is nothing like past, present, and future. The mind is conditioned by time, space, and causation, and meditation is the method of freedom from all these conditionings of the mind.

Remember the Center Within

Whenever you have time, sit down quietly, compose yourself, and just start remembering that the center deep down within you is beyond this thinking process of yours. Human beings cannot imagine anything higher or more abstract than themselves. The finest and the highest image that they can think of is their own image. Whenever they think of God, they think that God is a particular person. People think, "One day God is going to come down and give me enlightenment. I am preparing myself to see that particular great being called God." But in this way people only create a fantasy in their minds and start being dependent on a mere image. It may help them for a short while in some way or other, but this is not the way to freedom.

When we start knowing the Truth, when we start understanding the Reality within, then we come to know that worrying for happiness and peace and wisdom is very injurious. If we create a strong desire for peace and do not renounce that desire, then we will have no peace at all because there cannot be any peace, happiness, or wisdom as long as desire is there agitating our mind. We cannot experience anything of God if our mind remains agitated and dissipated by desires; we must first become calm, peaceful, and tranquil. Desire is the very root of all miseries. So we must become desireless by maintaining constant awareness of the here and now. To be desireless, we must always remember the center of consciousness within.

It is possible to achieve this awareness if you learn how to play your part in life. What is that part? To be calm, to be peaceful, to be happy. And then you will see your great capacity. By expanding your consciousness, by purifying your mind, action, and speech, you can slowly expand your capacity and attain the unknown.

To be able to do this, you must not allow desire to control your life. Being desireless does not mean that you should try not to eat or sleep, nor that you should refrain from using material things and living in the world. You should be free to do all things, but you should never allow worldly desires to delay your progress toward enlightenment. All worldly desires are mingled with sorrows. You should try to understand that those desires are dissipating your energy, and you should be fully aware of the purpose of life. You should learn to play your part while having constant awareness of the Reality and purpose within. You should allow all desires to be swallowed up by the one desire for attaining the higher purpose of life. Through this one highest desire you can direct your mind, speech, and action to desirelessness, which is the highest state of mind.

Ask for Nothing

It is desire that confines the mind and makes it small, selfish, conceited, and egotistical. When children build a house of sand, they think that it is very real, and they cannot be convinced otherwise. But reality eventually dawns, and they get tired of their make-believe and finally come to understand. Similarly, we perform many experiments to satisfy our desires by enjoying first this and then that particular object, but sooner or later we find that this is exactly like sucking the drops of water from a weed floating on the lake of life rather than drinking fully from the lake itself. It is not satisfying. Our desires are never satisfied but keep demanding more and more. Trying to satisfy our desires, or asking God to satisfy them, finally makes us weak and slavish. So be content; ask for nothing and you will receive that which is beneficial for you.

When we realize the Reality, asking is stopped and desires are ended. Then the mind is freed from its problems and conflicts. Such a mind is a fit instrument to help on the path of enlightenment. Have you ever, even for a second, realized a state of desirelessness? Just for a few seconds ask yourself not to have any desires. What will be the condition of your mind then? Immediately your mind will flow in an ocean of joy and bliss. When we are able to lead the mind to this state of desirelessness, then we are in a state of meditation. The purpose of meditation is to lead us to the highest state of desirelessness. There is a Persian story that explains this fact. It describes a swami who loved his practices, but one day he suddenly stopped praying, stopped repeating his mantra, stopped doing meditation. So people came to him and said, "Sir, what is this? You've been teaching us all our lives to do these things, but now we find that you no longer do any of them. What is the matter with you?" He replied, "When you pray for many things, you form the habit of asking, 'Give me this, give me that.' I have simply stopped all this asking, for I have at last come to know the Reality. What shall I ask for now? So I have stopped praying and asking God, 'Give me this, give me that.'"

The problem in trying to attain a peaceful mind is that no matter how hard we try, we find that from morning to night there is always a desire creeping into the mind. Desire is the motivation for all actions, speech, and emotions. There are a million desires, but hidden among them is this one small desire: "I wish I could see God." For most of us this is only a weak desire that is usually pushed aside by stronger, more powerful desires. But when the desire to know God is strengthened, it swallows all other desires, and finally this desire is fulfilled by attaining a height beyond itself called desirelessness.

When a swami renounces the world, he often acquires the desire for learning. He learns this thing and that, studies this book and that, but finally he finds that even the desire for learning is an obstacle for his highest attainment. Gandhi always said, "Reduce your desires to zero and you will have attainment." As long as you have any desires, you are tossed about and agitated in mind, and you are not at peace. But when you attain that center within through the practice of meditation, then you will have peace of mind.

Mantra, the Way to Peace

You must create the condition for the mind to be peaceful. To be peaceful means to have no desires. You must learn to say to all worries, desires, weaknesses, and temptations: "Leave me for a while; I will deal with you later on." It is necessary to have that determination before you sit to meditate; otherwise, all these desires will invade your mind during meditation. For example, normally you may be fairly happy, but when you sit to meditate you find that all the things you were supposed to do but put off now come to you and remind you of your duties. (You remember them because you are now directly in touch with that level of mind which holds the seeds of memory.) But if you sit down quietly and constantly remember your mantra for some time, you will find that for a few minutes you can really keep the mind busy with the mantra, and that during those moments you attain peace. Even if you do not consciously feel peaceful, by remembering your mantra you definitely receive subconscious peace, for you are constantly pouring the impression of your mantra into the subconscious mind. By implanting and strengthening the mantra, you are preparing the mind to help you when you are in need of help. This most important thing that we have kept within us will come to us when we are all alone. It is our very best friend in need.

The mantra is like a woman who wears a veil. Now, why does a woman wear a veil? She wants to not be seen by others, but only by her beloved. The mantra is exactly like that: it is useless for others who do not know what it is. It was not intended for them, but it is very powerful for the one for whom it was meant. The veil is intended for others, not for you yourself. You must totally unveil the mantra by constant repetition and use; it must carry you to the deepest level of life. First you repeat the mantra with your tongue; then you repeat it in your breath; next you remember it mentally. And then you hear your mantra with your whole being, as though your whole being is an ear and you are listening. But even this is not considered the highest state. The highest state of using the mantra is when the mantra starts absorbing the mind. The mantra eventually becomes an ocean of bliss in which the mind is floating.

In the beginning, the mantra will frequently be deflected by the mind. But when the mantra becomes established, when you receive its vibrations, when you really start feeling it, its effect is very strong. Your whole being absorbs the strength of the mantra, and you are transformed by it. You should try to understand and remember the strength within you. But that strength—the strength of the mantra and the teacher within—should never make you egotistical. That strength should transform your personality. That is called the divine strength within you. As you start turning inward, making your mind more subtle, then you will find that there is a center within you which will give you peace.

The Role of Women in Society

East/West Books, Chicago, Illinois, October 2, 1977

I want to remind the women of our age that they have forgotten their status. We are now passing through a difficult period. We want to have a glimpse of that civilization in which we can live with a sense of equality, loving all and excluding none, but in this search modern woman is forgetting her power within and forgetting a very important role that she has to play in society. If she doesn't play this role, there will be no happiness at all. If women want to bring a change in our society, they can definitely do it, because woman is the architect of our whole society and the architect of humanity's destiny. She built the home; she established the institution of family life; she brings up the children and makes them good citizens.

Do you know who first taught meditation in action? You may believe that it was Buddha, Krishna, or Christ, but actually the founders of meditation in daily life were women. In ancient India each woman in every village would go to the well in the evening to fetch water and to talk, gossip, or sing. Then as she came back to the village, she would balance her vessel of water on her head. She would carry the vessel on her head, with her arms at her side; she would never use her hands to hold the vessel steady. This requires tremendous concentration and control; even a great yogi may not be able to do such a thing. She might dance, even weep, and discuss various things with the other women, but that vessel would never fall. This is actually meditation in action. You can live in the world and yet remain above, exactly like that woman who has a water vessel on her head and yet does her duties without any problem and without being carried away from her center of concentration.

Shakti—the Female Power

Without woman, man is never complete. Tagore, a great Indian poet, has written, "O woman, you are half in reality but half in a dream." That dream which all men have, that dream without which humanity will not survive, that dream which is inexplicable, is really woman. She should try to understand her status in society. I have always considered women to be living temples. The most ancient scriptures say that without *shakti,* without the female power, it is not possible for humankind to survive. The female power has been the force behind all the great leaders of the world. For example, if you study the life of Ramakrishna Paramahansa, you will learn that he became great because of a woman. Likewise, Krishna became great because of Radha. And Buddha became great because of many women who played important roles in his life from the very beginning.

The problem regarding women today is not a matter of whether woman is higher or man is higher. As far as I am concerned, woman is definitely superior to man. If you put a man through a little discomfort, he will not easily tolerate it, but a woman comfortably lives with a baby in her womb, carrying it with her for many months, and then she goes through labor, which is like a death experience. Women alone have that capacity. They have the power of tolerance, endurance, and patience. Woman is both psychologically and medically superior to man. Very few women suffer heart attacks—because they are shock absorbers. They can go through pain easily, but when a man has a little bit of sneezing or pain he creates much fuss and carries on like a baby.

Women have the real strength, but the problem is that they are not making creative use of that strength. The world needs their help today. Woman is suffering because of her own lack of awareness of her strength. The power of shakti is being dissipated in advertising, playboy clubs, television programs, movies, magazines, books—and we are reaping the consequences. Women do not exist for the fun of men, but many women today have forgotten this. Many a woman is still looking for someone to appreciate her. I say, "Why do you want that? Why are you becoming dependent—wearing certain clothes and expecting a man to say that you look beautiful?" This way of life is not helpful for our rising generation. Women are also mothers, and such an attitude of dependence on men is not helpful for educating children. If we really love humanity, we should learn to understand this.

Custodians of Civilization

Women are the first teachers. Children receive their basic education from women. If a mother does not impart to the children the knowledge of how to live properly, they grow wild and always remain wild. But woman today is not secure. She is not sure that she is going to live in the same house or with the same man tomorrow. When the relationship is uncertain, she cannot properly impart knowledge to the child.

In India, the stability of women has been maintained, and we can learn from the results. India has gone through many, many tortures for two thousand years because of foreign rule. The last foreign rulers were English, so many Indians became psuedo-Britishers, wearing Western clothing and speaking English. Yet Indian culture and civilization survived. This happened not because of man, but because of woman. The custodians of Indian civilization and culture have always been women. The men came in touch with the alien rulers, but the women remained apart, and the alien rulers could not contact them. Thus, the culture and civilization remained intact. Everything crumbled except civilization. Today the material wealth of India is gone; there is poverty, disparity, malnutriton, and overpopulation—but there remains one thing: civilization. That ancient stream of civilization is still flowing freely in India because of women.

Fifty years ago, women in the West were also custodians of

civilization. But they are not custodians of culture today. Today there is no culture. There is no effective training in our present society. We create penitentiaries to control criminals, and we talk about therapy for the unhappy. But the main root for proper living is education in our childhood. The highest learning is not imparted in colleges or universities. "Be good, be kind, be gentle, don't be wild"—these principles are learned in childhood. Much of the education imparted in universities is not real education, but imitation; it is not satisfying to the human intellect and heart. Another kind of education is the environmental education that we receive from our friends, neighbors, and society. That is now also weak—because the foundation is not strong. The educational foundation is laid in childhood, and that totally depends on the mother. If our childhood education in the family is creative and productive, I don't think there will be any problem in society. We must learn to reconstruct that part of society, to rebuild that part of society which really forms the foundation of our lives.

We have been building many churches and educational institutions, but the main institution is the family. When it is ignored, we can never be happy. Dive into the heart of all problems, and you will discover that the base of all problems lies in the family life. If we do not appreciate the importance of the family, though our society may survive, it will create wild people with no understanding. So my first request to women is that instead of being preoccupied with whether they are inferior or superior to men, they reestablish the family life. Then there is a chance for future generations, a chance for the children to learn.

Yoga and Family Life

Himalayan Institute, Honesdale, Pennsylvania, April 19, 1980

The word yoga comes from the root *yug,* meaning "to unite."
There are various kinds of union. If you heat the two ends of a
single piece of metal and then join them together, they become as
one and form a ring. And when a man and a woman marry, they
exchange rings to symbolize their joining together as one. So
marriage, like yoga, means to unite, to join, to be one. In yoga, the
individual self becomes one with the universal Self. So the ultimate
goal of yoga and marriage is the same: to experience union, to
realize the reality which is called happiness. We are all here
because we have committed a mistake somewhere: we have
separated ourselves from the whole by feeding our egos. We can
regain the union we have lost, however. Even if we are physically
separate from the Reality, we can mentally regain it. In every walk
of life, with every step, we are constantly losing or gaining. Life is
like that. We can learn from both.

There are two ways to approach life: one is called renunciation and the other is called household life. There is only one
difference—on the path of renunciation there is more time to think
and understand, more time to teach. When I was a boy, whenever
I met those selfless wanderers in the mountains, they charmed me.
What a life! No responsibility. With only a blanket and a pot of
water, they wander from one mountain to another; they don't
know where they are going to spend the night, where they will eat,
or what they will eat. But in reality, renunciation is a very tough

89

path; it is not for everyone. Nor is a renunciate superior to those who live in the world. When a monk comes among you, you think he is greater than you. But if you are really doing your duty properly, he is not greater.

The role of most people is not to renounce. We can be one with the Reality another way—by doing our work, by discharging our duties, and by understanding something about life. In the path of action there are many means. We can apply all of them, and by so doing we can attain our goal. The first thing in both paths is the goal. We know many things, yet we know nothing. We are misled by our learning. We talk a lot about God, but no one knows what God is. Let us call God truth or ultimate happiness, for truth alone can make us happy. And that is the goal of both paths—happiness without an object. It is also called selfless love.

There is something the householder understands that the renunciate does not because the renunciate has not gone through the progression of life systematically. A householder wants to realize from the very beginning what love is, and he introduces himself to others through the body. In other words, you have a picture of yourself, and you say, "I look like this; I am different from you; I love you." You will find that as you come to understand love selflessly, you come to understand the meaning of life. As a householder, you are making an experiment, and there are various ways of doing it. For the majority of people, family life is like a fortress. Those who are inside do not know how to come out of it; those who are out are pushing to get in. It should not be like that. Family life should be like a Garden of Eden where we can live and enjoy ourselves and be happy.

Love Means Expanding Yourself

The real aim of life is to understand love, but most people never learn this. When two people get together they are charmed by each other, but the time comes when they cannot adjust, and then they separate; they get scared and think the relationship of marriage is not a healthy thing. That is not true. The problem is that the way one is thinking, the other is not thinking; they think in entirely different ways. And then there is conflict, clash. And if they go on creating conflicts, these conflicts become the source of disease and misery. So don't allow conflict in your daily life. Let us explore and find out how to lead a good life, a happy life, for if two people have the right understanding—if two people are compatible, not only on the physical level, but with understanding—then they can be very happy and do tremendous work in the world.

The most ancient traveler in the world is called love. Even before this earth came into existence, that omnipotent and omniscient power called truth expanded to create the universe because of love. Love means expansion. And then there is its opposite, called hatred or contraction. Watch what happens some day when you start hating somebody—when someone is not doing what you want, is not fulfilling your expectations. You contract your personality, you isolate yourself. So there are two laws of life: the law of expansion, and the law of contraction. When we are under the law of contraction, we squeeze ourselves so much that we lose our identity. Our personality and character change; our whole being changes by hating, by not understanding the principle of expansion.

Everyone lives in two worlds, not just one. We cannot maintain our existence if we do not understand that we are citizens of two worlds—the world within and the world outside. The best human being is the one who creates a bridge between the inner and outer worlds; for if we are not happy within ourselves, we cannot make others happy. To make others happy, we have to be happy—and we cannot be happy if we follow the law of contraction, withdrawal, egotism. Many of us have the problem that we spend our whole life trying to undo something that happened in our childhood—and so we don't go anywhere, we don't progress in life. Instead of doing this, we have to learn to be generous; we have to expand ourselves.

Childhood is very important. Those who are mothers, and those who want to be mothers, should understand that no society was ever built by man. Whatever there is was built by woman. Women are the builders. Man has been a barbarian—irresponsible throughout history. It is woman who has built society. But today woman too has become irresponsible. She chooses to have a career and leaves the baby with a babysitter. Children should not lose their training ground. That is very important. The more attention you pay to your child, the more the child will grow. Attention is the key point in daily life. Nothing can exist without attention. Certain seeds are sown in childhood, and they are very strong. All the gems of truth are taught in childhood. So as a parent, be kind, be good, be loving, be gentle. Remember that the aim of life is to understand love—and that means expanding yourself.

Family life can teach you without "learning"; you can learn without formal instruction or study. It is a daily experience. You don't need to read a book on how to love your husband or how to love your child. You can get suggestions from others about how to take care of your child, but you don't need to learn from anybody else how to love it. Even the newborn baby knows where to get milk. Put it near its mother's body and the baby goes toward the breast. Who teaches it? Who teaches animals? How do they know? How does that little baby know where the breast is? We all have something that is called instinct. It is natural, and in human beings instinct is refined: it goes down deep to the center of consciousness, which is called intuition. That is why we are considered to be superior to other creatures. We can express ourselves—and if we learn to express ourselves with love, life can be happy.

The Journey of Love and Life

The belief that if we do not have something we will be unhappy is a myth, but most of us live by that myth. We say, "I don't have a good car or a job, therefore I am unhappy" or "I don't have a good house or a husband or a wife, so I am unhappy." That is not the way to live, yet what do we do? Our whole life we involve ourselves with our families and with collecting things, but we are still unhappy because we are not aware of one fact: all the objects around us are only the means. They are not the goal: happiness is the goal. We have to supply the means to make ourselves happy.

A child is the means to complete your relationship. Two people are in love, and they get married. Their love travels to deeper levels, and a child is born. Still they are not complete; they want an education for the child. They see the child growing, and the child does not stop growing at any certain point—he or she goes on. So the child gets more education and grows to maturity. But this does not fulfill another part of the parents' life—internal growth. So their love travels in other directions, and their consciousness starts expanding toward something higher. Love travels more. What is love? Traveling. What is life? Traveling. It is not a pool of stagnation. It is traveling. But most people create a pool of stagnation and call it love. They call it family life, but it is not. Family life is meant to radiate love to others. We are not meant to be jealous or mean or bad to our neighbors. The whole purpose of building the small world called family life is lost when you think like that. "I have a child, so I should be very greedy," you think, but this will not help you. "I have a child, so I should be afraid of the future." That will not help you either; that is being selfish.

A new husband and wife can get together on a sensual level, but they do not yet know the other joy—how to be selfless. So nature says, "I am going to help you. You will have a child." When a child is born, many fathers become selfish and move to another room. "The child is disturbing me," they say. Then the second step comes when the father thinks that his wife is paying too much attention to their child and not enough to him. "Perhaps she loves the child more than me," he thinks. Many mean thoughts start arising in his mind because he has not learned how to be selfless. Whenever you are selfish, remember that your growth is stunted. Whenever you are selfless, remember that you are growing. Family life is a field for experiments on how to expand. First you love your husband or wife; then love goes to your children; then it goes to your children's friends; then it goes to your neighbors; and it goes on expanding like this. Love and life and expansion are all one and the same. So learn to be as selfless as you can from the very beginning. It will help you.

Yoga tells us how we can be selfless by learning to control the fluctuations of our mind. Control means directing those faculties; it does not mean stopping them. Suppose you are a newly married couple, and I tell you that you should control your sexual life. What do I mean by that? I mean, do not be so involved in sexual life that you don't think about anything except sex. Don't do that. If you do, you will lose respect, reverence, and love for sexual life. So first of all, do not overdo. Observe your capacity; observe your strength and understanding. This is called control. The first lesson yoga teaches is to observe, to understand, to be aware of our whole strength—and strength comes from within. The so-called comforts of life can temporarily make us happy and momentarily inspire us, but ultimately they cannot do this. Ultimately we need inner strength, which we have to build slowly in daily life. Why do a wife and husband love each other and yet separate? Because they have not made experiments; they have not adjusted; they have not developed inner strength.

Strength Resides Within

Human beings are fully equipped to develop their strength if they would only tap the source of knowledge within themselves. As strong as we are outside, we have more than a million times that strength inside. Did you ever try to tap it? That strength is within us. A huge rock does not have the strength that is found in a molecule, in an atom, in a subatomic particle—and when we split that particle, we will find even more strength. In the same way, if we go to deeper levels, we will find more and more strength within ourselves. Do you ever use that strength in a creative way? How much time do you waste in your daily life with useless worry? Worry and negativity take up most of your time. "What will happen if I die?" you think. "What will happen if I have an accident or get sick?" "What will happen if my wife leaves me?" "What will happen if my husband leaves?" What type of love is this? You are both insecure, thinking all the time that either one of you might leave the other. Many poets say that in deep love we are always insecure, but that is not deep love. If you are insecure in your love, you do not really love the other person.

The best way to find happiness is not to listen to the disciplines imposed on you by others but to get into a program of self-discipline. It does not matter how many times you fail—just make a sincere effort. But all discipline should be based on two points: that your goal is happiness, and that you will apply everything you have toward gaining it. Any skill you have will help you in attaining your goal. In addition, all that you know about good food, good exercise, a good way of breathing, a good way of cooking your food, a good way of leading your sexual life, can be a means for achieving it. The best way, however, is to have reverence for your partner. In a relationship it is very important not only to love, but also to have reverence toward the one you love, for if you do not respect your love, it is a mockery; it is selfishness. On the ladder of love, the first step is reverence for your partner. If you do not have that, you will be finding fault all the time. "You always do this," you will say. "You do not do this; you have not done that." Adjustment, on the other hand, leads to a state of fulfillment. So you should not be in competition.

Many times I have said to someone that his wife was a good person, and he has not liked it. He says, "What about me?" He doesn't understand what I am trying to tell him. If someone is praising your wife, you should be very happy. I can easily find out about your love for your wife by praising her and watching your face. Your expression is a measure of your love for your wife. Then I tell her, "I met your husband, and he is a very good person." If you are not happy when someone admires your wife or children, if you are only happy when someone admires you, it means that you have not learned to respect the relationships you have, to admire, to have reverence for them.

It is a great thing when two people decide to attain one goal—happiness. That is something great, and if they make an effort, they can be successful. They don't need any advisor to counsel them; they should thrash out their own problems by being kind, gentle, good, loving, patient, and tolerant. All they need is a little self-control, a little restraint, and some understanding. It would be easier if people did not go so fast when they get together. Why not understand this point from the beginning? Men and women are not objects; they are living beings that radiate love. If they have love, they give love. They should not treat one another as objects. If something happens to an object, or if part of it does not function properly, we try to replace it. But we cannot do that with human beings.

Express Love on Three Levels

We can express our love in many ways. When someone is sick, for instance, we can show our love for that person more than at any other time by caring for her or him. We can express love through mind, speech, and action, but many people do not communicate with their loved ones on all these levels. Sometimes a husband is outwardly very nice to his wife, but mentally he is not. He does not respect her; he does not love her. He is a good provider, but he is not a good husband. So we should learn to communicate on all three levels.

When there is a newborn baby, the wife and husband often go through many hassles and problems. The husband says, "You are paying so much attention to the child. You don't love me any more." The wife says, "The child belongs to both of us and needs care." The wife is not capable of satisfying her husband's sexual needs during these days. He feels rejected—he should not, but because he is selfish, he does. So the child has bad dreams; its body jerks; it is unhappy because of the parents' thoughts and feelings. This is a fact. And even if the parents fight quietly, it will still affect the child. The baby will toss and turn and not get enough rest. It may even have bad digestion. In this way, the child is showing them that they are doing something that is against the law of love. And they are hurting themselves as well as the poor innocent child.

Family life is not a simple responsibility; it is not a simple commitment; it is not a simple commandment. It can be a great joy, provided you know how to express yourself through the mind as well as through action and speech. In other words, to fully enjoy life, to be successful, you should learn to use your mind. If it is going toward negativity, you and your partner can never meet, so mentally you should learn to be positive all the time. "I can do it," you should say. "I will be able to do it, and I will do it." This is positive feedback that you can give to your mind. If we are positive, our expressions, our actions, and our speech will be positive too. But if our mind is not positive, we cannot take positive action.

So do not reject each other, and do not absorb each other's individuality or try to create dependency. That is not love; that is not the right way of doing things. Remain independent and do not make your partner or anyone else dependent. A wife and husband should remain independent but together; they should be mentally positive, not negative; and they should not be passive, for passivity means giving up. Overconfidence is also not good. That will not lead to success in family life. We should be confident, we should be self-reliant, but that comes when we have a realistic understanding of ourselves and our abilities.

Failure should not make us negative. One's whole life is an experiment in trying to find happiness; it is not necessary that we have success all the time. Divers search in the ocean for pearls; they don't find them every time. They may have to dive twenty or thirty times in the deep sea to get them—and even then they don't always succeed. Sometimes they may not find certain pearls for years, although the pearls are there. The diver is doing his duty, but he is not getting a reward. Each of us must likewise make repeated efforts in our own life. Always make an effort. But there should be sincerity in it.

We should learn to talk with each other. If we shoot someone, the bullet can be taken out and the body may heal, but if we speak a harsh word, it can never be recalled. It can do far more damage than a bullet. For instance, suppose a man loves his wife, but one day he loses his temper and swears at her. She will never forget it. Why did he do it? Because it was already in his mind. Therefore, watch yourself to see how much you bottle up. Watch for the reasons you do not speak up. On the other hand, do not fight. Do not try to disperse things in one word. Relax. Listen to what the other wants. Say, "I don't like to fight. Whatever you say, I will try to understand; whatever I say, you will try to understand." Don't keep telling the other, "You are doing this; you are doing that; you are not doing this." Allow your partner to find out for herself or himself; let your partner see how much capacity she or he has.

Not all subjects should be discussed before going to bed or before taking food. Try to be positive then—even if you have been negative the whole day. It will help you. On the other hand, if you are positive the whole day but are negative these two times, it will hurt your family life. There should be understanding between you and your partner, and there should also be time. There should be one day a week that is completely devoted to the relationship, a day that has no other purpose in it. Once a week, one day should be given to your partner. You can say, "Let us speak of everything we have not said. This does not mean that either of us has to accept everything the other says. Just listen, and I will also." A woman is not a piece of furniture that can be replaced, and a man should not be accepted or used as a visitor. If they respect their love, a man and a woman can lead a very good life together and attain their goal of happiness. Yoga says that by doing your duty selflessly and skillfully, you can attain your goal here in this lifetime. It can be done.

So communicate with your partner on three levels—mind, speech, and action. If you want to make yourself happy, learn that you have to make the people with whom you live happy. Pay attention to the things you are doing. In this way, you are training yourself. Do not forget your goal. Negativity and passivity are not going to help you. Learn that life is expansion, not contraction. Don't go toward egotism. Learn to expand, and in this way you will grow by giving, giving, giving. Please grow with love in this life.

Keys to Successful Living

Himalayan Institute, Glenview, Illinois, June 6, 1982

Everyone wants to be successful in life, but where are the keys to success? Do we have to go out and search for those keys, or do we have those potentials already within ourselves? When we begin to examine life, we can see that it is divided into two aspects—life within and life without; internal life and external life—and we can see that these aspects are of equal importance. Even if we have renounced the world, gone far away from civilization, and live in the wilderness doing nothing but meditation, we cannot ignore external life. We still have to see that we eat, do our ablutions, and perform our practices on time. So life in the external world is as important as life in the internal world. Even one who has renounced the world has to understand the word *relationship* properly, because life itself is actually relationship. The body is related to the breath, and the breath is related to the mind. The body, breath, senses, and mind all function together as a unit. So life virtually means relationship, and thus the art of living and being requires an understanding of one's relationship to the external world and the relationships within oneself.

All human beings have inner potentials, but many people are not aware of those potentials and do not know how to use them to have a successful life. Those who are not happy internally can never be happy externally; those who are not happy within themselves can never make others happy. Those who do not love themselves can never love others.

If we are not happy, how can we be successful in life? Success lies in our happiness. The keys to happiness lie within us, but our modern education does not teach us how to find them. It is helpful to have a few formulas to practice in daily life to make it more successful. I have not created these formulas; they are derived from observations based on experience. There are five points to remember: first, how to decide things on time; second, how to study personal habit patterns; third, how to conduct ourselves in the external world; fourth, what attitude to take; fifth, where to find happiness. To attain success in life, one should learn and apply these five points.

Deciding Things on Time

The first point to understand is the philosophy and science of decision—how to make decisions on time. The most successful person is that person who knows how to decide on time. There are many extraordinarily brilliant people who understand things very quickly, but when the time comes to make a decision, when an opportunity comes, they withdraw and are not able to act. They do not know how to decide. They know they should learn to decide on time, but they don't do it. They always say, "Well, I knew it. I understood the key, but I did not act in time." Though they may think correctly, and accurately understand the situation properly, they suddenly lose confidence. This is a world of competition; someone else is always trying to attain the same thing we are. So if we do not decide on time, someone else will attain what we want. Time is valuable in the external world. A tender bamboo can be easily bent, but if we try to bend a mature bamboo, it will break. That which we have to do today, we should not postpone for tomorrow, but we should also not make decisions in haste.

We may have a setback if we make a wrong decision, but our mistakes will teach us. Many people avoid making decisions their whole lives, so their decisive faculty of mind, the faculty of discrimination, becomes rusty and dies. Such people become totally dependent on others. When we study the four functions of the mind—*buddhi*, the faculty of decisiveness; *ego*, the principle of identity; *chitta*, the storehouse of impressions; and *manas*, the importer and exporter of sensations and experience—then we become aware of the power of the will. Will power is that something within us that comes forward and says, "Do this. It will be helpful for you." Training the internal functions helps us to understand the decisive faculty of the mind, without which we cannot be successful.

We should understand our capacities and potentials, and then we should express ourselves in the external world with full confidence, acting without any reservations. Thus there are three steps in performing an action: first, forming an opinion within ourselves; second, expressing our opinion to others; and third, executing our opinion in action.

Understanding Habit Patterns

The main thing that one should learn in life—and it is not taught in the home or in the schools—is self-analysis. We should learn to analyze ourselves. If we really want to understand ourselves, we can analyze our personality by understanding our habit patterns. This is not difficult. We should simply try to be consciously aware of every action we perform and realize that our actions are virtually our thoughts. Without thought there can be no action. Habit patterns and thoughts are revealed through behavior.

There is a branch of psychology called behaviorism that is based on this concept. But one should understand that external behavior alone cannot reveal everything about a person. Laughter, for example, cannot be analyzed behaviorally. If I were to laugh, you might also laugh with me simply because I was laughing but without understanding why I was laughing. Your laughter is out of sheer reaction. Then you might laugh a second time, this time at yourself because you did not understand why you were laughing and yet you laughed. You might also laugh a third time because you finally understand what I was laughing at and you now also find it funny. All three times your laughter might seem the same to others, but each time it had a different motivation. So internal states cannot be understood through behavior analysis alone. Only a small part of oneself and others can be understood through observing behavior. But knowing our habit patterns can help us to analyze and understand our personality.

What is personality? The word "personality" comes from the root *persona*, which means "mask." Our personality is a mask that we wear. We don't have to wear a mask when we are by ourselves; we wear a mask to express ourselves to others. Our personality is a character, and that character is composed of certain habits. Each of us has numerous habits; so when we want to understand our personality, we should understand our habit patterns. A habit pattern is a conscious thought or action that one repeats again and again. This creates a groove in the unconscious mind and forms an unconscious habit. Unconscious habits are stronger than conscious habits. All habit patterns are self-created. When we sit down and try to understand which of our habits control our life, we see that there are many deep-rooted habits within us. We should learn to study them. Once we become aware of harmful thoughts and emotions that have created deep grooves in the mind, we can begin to change them by creating new grooves. Then the mind will stop flowing to the old grooves and start flowing to the new ones. In this way we can change our habits.

You should also learn to execute your intentions. For instance, many people have very good intentions to do something nice for their neighbors, and they think about it all the time, but then those thoughts are never executed, they are never allowed to become actions. We have many thoughts that have never been executed, and that is why we are miserable. If we learn to select those thoughts that are helpful and then allow ourselves to execute them, that brings fulfillment, and life will be happy. We create misery for ourselves when we do not bring our good thoughts into action. One of the French writers has explained this concept beautifully: "All good thoughts that are not brought into action are either treachery or abortion." Good thoughts are those that help others and that help us also. Bad thoughts are those that obstruct our progress and create barriers for others.

Deep-seated habits can keep you from doing that which you know would be good for you to do. You become helpless because of the obsessions and addictions that are caused by your habits. You may continue in a habit that you know is not good—that is neither healthy nor helpful and that should not be done—because the habit has become so deep-rooted that you are powerless to change your behavior. Society does not help you change your bad habits, and there are very few places where you can get help. Many people who are in the penitentiary know that what they have done is a crime, but the force of habit led them to act improperly. Their faculty of discrimination within functions—they understand what is right and what is not right—but their deep-seated habits have motivated them to do something that is not good, that is not acceptable. Actually, no one should be considered either a good person or a bad person. In traditional English law, when someone was punished, he was told, "We are not punishing you for yourself. We are punishing you for your bad habits."

Controlling the Primitive Urges

Habit patterns are very strong motivations in life; we should not ignore them. We should not create a defense mechanism and say, "Well, so what if I have this habit?" We should learn to study our habit patterns and work with our habits to change them. There are very few basic habits, and they arise from four fountains: food, sex, sleep, and self-preservation. By understanding these four primitive fountains, we can understand our habit patterns, and then we can learn to change them and to transform the personality.

Food is the first basic urge. If a husband tells his wife, "Don't overeat," she may say, "I overeat because of you. You don't pay attention to me, so I have to overeat." Sometimes when the sexual appetite is not dealt with properly, people overeat. This is the universal law of compensation. If we maintain a nutritious diet, we will not have any problem from the primitive fountain called food.

Food goes through the body and then affects the mind, but sex originates in the mind and then is expressed through the body. If our mind is balanced and we have attained emotional maturity, then we can deal competently with the sex urge. For it is the mind, not the body, that deals with sex. The poor body cannot handle the rush, the flood, of mind, and so almost no one is sexually happy. To have a balanced sex life, one should understand that a calm, tranquil mind is very helpful.

Sleep is another primitive fountain. We consider ourselves to be extremely knowledgeable and highly advanced, but we do not know anything about how to sleep. It is very important to understand the anatomy of sleep. If you wanted to go to sleep right now, you could not do it because you need many accomodations to create the proper atmosphere for sleep, but yogis know how to go to sleep voluntarily, remain conscious, and then wake up at the exact moment they had determined they would. People go to sleep just out of habit, but we should learn to train our will so we can go to sleep or wake up anytime we want to. And when we sleep, we should be conscious. This is possible. There are methods for going to deep sleep, recording what is going on around us, and then waking up and remembering it. Yogis know these methods and have demonstrated them scientifically. People do not need to sleep as much as they are in the habit of doing. We can go to the state of deep sleep for just two hours and awaken totally refreshed. This has been observed by scientists who have done research on the anatomy of sleep. If we know how to sleep, we can give complete rest to the body and to the conscious mind anytime.

The fourth fountain is self-preservation. Fear comes from the urge for self-preservation, and when fears are deepened, they create phobias. People are always trying to protect themselves; they are always afraid. It is good to protect ourselves from the physical world, but it is not good to protect ourselves from the mental world—that is very dangerous. People should learn to face their inner fears and to understand why they are afraid. People always want to avoid unpleasant things, and so they never examine their fears. That is why they have innumerable fears within them. Most fears are unexamined, and they are imaginary; they are not valid. "My husband has not come home. Perhaps he has had an accident. Perhaps something awful has happened!" Why imagine only the negative; why not imagine the positive also? "My husband has not come home. Perhaps he has won the lottery today. Perhaps he has become a millionaire!" People are in the habit of creating imaginary fears, and when they don't come true, they forget them. They don't go back and analyze those fears. Even when people know that their fear is imaginary, that self-created fear still makes them miserable.

Even when people are in love, they are afraid of the beloved. "Perhaps she is angry. Perhaps I have done something wrong and made her unhappy." People are also always afraid of their enemies. People form a strong habit of being afraid of everything. But when they learn to examine their fears, they realize that all fears are imaginary. Imaginary means there is an image within. We receive an image from outside, from our relationship, and then we create an image within; we have millions of images within us. To be free from all fears, we must learn to face fearsome images and to examine them. Fears are extremely dangerous, but they are all self-created. Learning to live free from the fears that arise from the urge of self-preservation is very important.

Living in the External World

How can one live successfully in the external world? It is very difficult to live in the external world, to put up with the world, to deal with the whims of many people, to please everyone. So it is helpful to have a few principles to apply to the various situations and circumstances we find ourselves involved in. Then alone is it possible for us to be successful. We have numerous experiences every day—some pleasant, some unpleasant. But there is one category of experience for which we long: the kind of experience that guides us, that motivates us to do something helpful for others and for ourselves. But such experiences are very rare.

We waste our time and energy. Even the time and energy that we think we are spending in pleasure we do not enjoy, because we do not really know how to enjoy the things of the world. But we can learn how to do this; all the things of the world can be enjoyed. The renunciates say, "Your world does not have anything. It's not a good world. All things are fleeting, all things are changing. All things are momentary, and nothing makes you happy. Why are you in this world? Why do you not renounce?" But they are wrong. We can live in the world and learn to use the things of the world as means. As St. Bernard says, "Learn to use the things of the world, but love God alone." The things of the world should not be loved. Their nature should be understood, and they should become means, but they should not be loved. When we use them, we tend to get attached to them—that is not healthy. We should love God alone, and we should learn that all the things of the world are to be used solely as means for attaining the center of love. The Lord of life is called love. We should learn to love our responsibilities and to discharge our duties lovingly, without any attachment.

Western students think that it is not possible to love someone without attachment. But perhaps the word attachment is not understood. Love is different from attachment. In love we give— we do our duties lovingly—and that is entirely different from attachment. Attachment is unauthorized. In attachment we become blindfolded and selfish. In attachment we expect all the time and we are never fulfilled, and thus we become miserable. There is not one single thing that we can say is really ours. We can have things—and we should learn to look after them properly— but we should not try to possess them. In attachment people are afraid. "This is mine. What will happen to me if it dies? What will happen to me if it is destroyed?" People remain constantly under the pressure of the fear of losing what they have or of not gaining what they want. The whole problem of fear arises from these two sources.

Most people are not aware that they are on a voyage. They are in the habit of collecting useless garbage, and it creates problems for them. People should learn to understand that needs and necessities are different from wants and desires. If we need something, we should have it, but we should not uselessly want to have unnecessary things. In studying the lives of great people, we find they share one trait that has made them successful: they do not take what they do not need. Once when Buddha was going as usual from door to door with his begging bowl to beg for alms, a housewife shouted at him, "You idiot! You are so healthy, so strong, and so handsome. You were a prince! Why did you renounce your home and start troubling us? Every day you come with your begging bowl. It has become too much for us." She was very angry because the whole city was full of renunciates, and there were very few householders; it was a problem for the householders to feed all the monks. She became so angry that she picked up some filth and tried to give it to him. He smiled and said, "Mother, I don't need it." He started to go on his way, but one of his disciples got angry and told the woman, "I am going to kill you for behaving like this with my Lord!" Buddha turned back to him and said, "You are not my disciple. You have not learned anything from me. If somebody wants to give you something undesirable, don't take it. If somebody says you are bad, don't accept such a negative suggestion." We should learn to understand this point, and then we can go through the process of life unaffected.

But instead of remaining unaffected, people allow their cultural values to make them dependent on external suggestions. We are blasted by suggestions all the time, and the power of suggestion is immense. If ten people say that we look ill, then we begin to feel sick. If someone says "You ugly person," then your whole day is ruined. But if someone says "Oh, you look beautiful!" then you say "You have made my day." You are already beautiful, but if nobody appreciates you, you don't believe in your beauty. You should learn to appreciate and admire yourself; you should learn to understand and come in touch with that beauty which is within you all the time. You are already beautiful just as you are! You do not need others to tell you you are beautiful. You should not become dependent on others' opinions; you should not try to know yourself through others.

There is a very dangerous characteristic in this culture: people make themselves dependent on each other. People live on suggestions; they are swayed by whatever anyone says. People are in the habit of always wanting and expecting attention from others, and this is very dangerous, because then life becomes totally dependent on others. This is the worst trait I have seen in Western culture. Wives nag their husbands and husbands criticize their wives because they expect too much from each other. When people become dependent on their relationships, when they expect too much from their relationships, then they are bound to suffer.

When a girl goes to school, the thought that constantly lives in her mind is that she will meet a good boy, get married, and be happy. But there is no Bible in the world that says marriage will make someone happy. Marriage does not make anyone happy; it is only a means for happiness in life, and if this is understood, then it is very good. But if one expects too much and thinks that marriage is the answer to all the vital questions of life, then that person will find only disappointment. People grow up with unreal expectations about marriage, and the philosophy of marriage is not taught. What is the purpose of marriage? What is the philosophy of remaining single? If a single person does not know how to use his time positively, and if he has no personal philosophy of life, then he becomes perverted. Those who are unmarried are not happy, and those who are married are also not happy. Marriage is like a fortress: those who are inside cannot come out, and those who are outside are rushing to get in. So I have not seen anyone who is happy. This does not mean that people should not get married; the institution of marriage is very necessary. If it crumbles, all of society will crumble. This is a great discipline for human society.

Developing the Proper Attitude

What should our attitude in the world be? It should be that relationships and all the things of the world are means. The world has never given anyone enlightenment, but at the same time it is impossible for one to get enlightened if one does not live in the world. What helplessness! The world does not give enlightenment, and yet we have to live in the world. Therefore let us understand that the world should be a means for enlightenment. There are two ways of using the world for this purpose: first, you can have the attitude that you will not allow the world to disturb you, so that you can thereby get enlightenment; and second, you can have the attitude that you can use the world to help you, so that you can thereby get enlightenment. Both attitudes should be applied. One should have the same attitudes toward relationships: "I will behave in such a way with my spouse and children that they don't disturb my inner peace; I will behave in such a way that they become helpful to me and that they also grow."

You should first have the attitude that no matter what happens, you will not be disturbed. Otherwise, when you get something, you become emotional and imbalanced, and when you don't get something, you become depressed and disorganized. This means that you do not have the proper attitude behind your thinking and behavior. Great leaders like Moses and Jesus had to face many serious problems, but they had the proper attitude. That attitude can be built only when you consider all relationships in the external world and all the objects of the world simply as means, not ends. Then it doesn't matter if today you expect something to become your means, and tomorrow you see that it will not. When your attitude toward the external world is that all the things of the world are means, and not disturbances, then you can find happiness.

Where Is Happiness?

If happiness were external, Americans would have it. Americans have many things, but they are not happy. Many people are very nice to others, but they are not nice to themselves. They have a mechanical way of behaving nicely with others, but they do not know how to be happy within themselves. They are creating a great conflict, a split personality, by pretending to express a happiness that is not there. Happiness is not in the external world; it is not attained through objects. People spend their whole lives wanting to have this and have that; they love objects, and they cannot love without objects. But the day you learn to love without an object, that will be the day of greatest happiness. When one learns to love God, that is love without an object. God is not an object; God is beyond all objects. So love without an object is love for God.

Happiness lies within you, and you should learn to use all things and apply all means to attain that happiness. This inner happiness is in a dormant form; you have to unfold yourself to experience it. Therefore you should learn to be still, so that the godly part in you can reveal itself to you. "Be still and know that I am God." What a great promise! This is the greatest aphorism. Many Christians and Jews think that there is no meditation in the Bible, but this one sentence reveals the entire philosophy of meditation.

Every human being should learn to be calm and quiet, and to see God in others. Then you can be detached from the nongodly part, and you will be loving the godly part. You are a shrine of God. I should love you because I should love God in you. It's good to love people because everyone is a temple of God. People do not worship the walls of a temple; their love is directed toward that which dwells inside it. So whomever you love, love God in that person.

I pray to the divinity within you.

Self-Analysis and Self-Enlightenment

Himalayan Institute, Glenview, Illinois, May 23, 1982

We think that the word "self" means only the body, senses, breath, and mind because we do not know that which supports the body, senses, breath, and mind. By understanding the nature of these aspects of the self, we can realize that which is the real support behind them.

We have a body, and it is a compound of five elements, or *tattvas*—earth, water, fire, air, and space. But we are not the body; the body is but a garment. How much time do we waste in looking after this garment, while the other levels of our life go ignored? We have this garment called the body, but we are sensing beings also. We have ten senses: five senses of cognition—smelling, tasting, touching, seeing, hearing—and five senses of action—mouth to eat, hands to work, legs to walk, and the two gates of elimination. These ten senses function because they are employed by the mind to express oneself in the external world. We think, and then we act; the body moves according to our thinking and feeling. So we are not only physical beings, we are thinking beings too, and when we study our thinking process we realize that it has various aspects or faculties, which in yoga are called modifications of the mind. Among all the faculties of the mind, four are considered to be very important: *buddhi*, the intellect; *manas*, the sensory-motor mind; *ahankara*, the ego; and *chitta*, the bed of memory through which consciousness flows directly from its source. That source is called the center of consciousness, the individual Self. Consciousness is the finest of all energies, and the flow of that energy motivates the

111

mind. This diagram will help you to understand the subject matter being discussed:

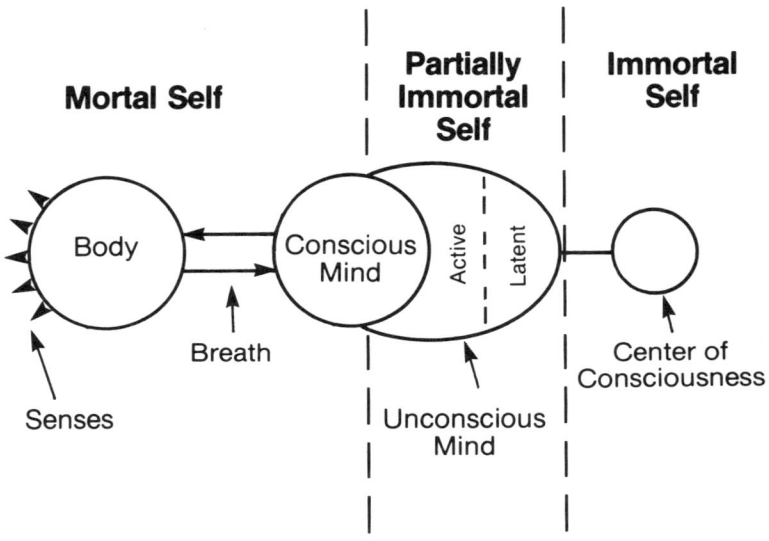

Breath—the Link

Between the body and the mind there is a link, and without that link, the body and mind cannot exist or function together. That link is called the breathing process. The day a person stops breathing, the body separates from the mind, and death occurs. This link—the breath—is very interesting and instructive. We can learn something about life just by observing how we are breathing. It is not necessary to study any books about the anatomy of breath to learn this. There are gases—such as carbon dioxide, oxygen, and nitrogen—without which we cannot live. But if someone simply pumps all of these gases into a person's body, he will not be able to survive. There is something deeper than mere gases that sustains life, and yoga literature terms this force *prana*. Prana is more subtle than breath; breath is the vehicle that supplies prana, the vital energy, to our system.

Inhalation and exhalation, or *prana* and *apana*, are two vehicles that constantly serve the city of life. Prana is called the supplier of energy, and apana is called the fire of death. Prana supplies energy through the liver, heart, brain, and spleen, and apana cleanses through the pores, lungs, kidneys, and bowels. No matter who you are—whether you are a sage, a criminal, a president, or a pauper—these two vehicles are always serving you. Whether you are waking, sleeping, or dreaming; whether you are absent-minded or fully alert; whether you are a woman, a man, or a child—prana and apana are constantly functioning.

What is that element inside us that regulates these two vehicles? Who is supplying that life breath, and who is receiving it inside? There is a particular branch of yogis called *Pranavedins* ("knowers of prana") who explain this. They do not identify themselves with any sect or religion but accept only the philosophy of prana. They say, "Our philosophy is complete. It is a practical philosophy, but other philosophies are based on imagination and speculation." They say that the one who is supplying energy to all is the Lord of everyone's life, that there is only one proprietor of all these bodies, and if He refuses to supply the energy, these bodies will all crumble. The universal Lord is supplying energy to the Lord of each individual body. On one end of the line is the universal Lord, and on the other end is that which we are. We are no different from that universal, cosmic energy; there is no difference at all. The Pranavedins say that their philosophy is concrete because they can catch the breath as it flies to where the center of consciousness is hidden. They say, "We can easily go to that center. Your philosophies, your religions, your rituals are all impractical."

There are very few sages who know this subject, but for those who really know it, pain, misery, and even death are nothing. They say, "We know what death means; we know what birth means. One who knows how to die also knows how to be born." So birth and death are completely under their conscious control. I have met a few of these sages, and I was in training with them for many years. They would leave their bodies aside, and if you examined one of these bodies scientifically, you would know that it was lifeless. But then they would return again, and their bodies would function as before. In the same manner, they would leave their bodies and get into other bodies and start walking and functioning naturally. This is a very advanced stage, and it is not possible for a common human being to do all this because it requires complete dedication, devotion, and self-surrender to the science of prana. The Pranavedins devote all their time and energy to knowing these *kriyas*, or methods. They say that because the mind cannot function without the vital force, prana is even superior to the functioning of the mind.

Mind—the Creator

The first layer of a human being is the body, the second is prana or vital energy, the third is the mind. There are two compartments of thinking: one is called the conscious mind, and the other is called the unconscious mind. The unconscious mind is a vast reservoir into which we continuously pour all the things we do—all our memories of the past, all our imaginings of the future, and everything we are doing in the present. Anything we have sensed, imagined, or thought makes an impression in the storehouse of the unconscious mind.

There is no educational program anywhere in the world that helps train the unconscious mind, that teaches how to have control over the unconscious and then go beyond. Only a very small part of us, the conscious mind, is being trained by our so-called educational system, so we have to train ourselves. We suffer because we do not know how to utilize the energy, the resources, that are already within us. Our problem is not the lack of resources; it is the way we think. We have all the resources, but we do not know how to utilize them to attain the purpose of life.

The purpose of life is not to attain God; it is to attain a state of mind that is free from all pains and miseries. That state which is free from all pains and miseries is a state of happiness, and that happiness bestows bliss and wisdom. An accurate analysis of the individual self can give you freedom from many problems. For who has created the problems human beings suffer from? Religion leads people to believe that God did, and if all the followers of religion suddenly ceased to accept this answer, everything would crumble: the structure of society and the formulas that people have made for themselves—and particularly for others—would completely crumble. Their values for deciding that this person is good and that person is bad—all this would crumble. But, actually, it is not God who makes someone good and someone else bad. Who, then, is responsible for doing this? The mind, with the help of the senses. The mind is a creator that makes something out of nothing; it creates fantasies. The world has not been created by God; the world has been manifested by God. All these faces belong to God; this is all his manifestation. All problems, all miseries, all pains, are created by the mind. When we create miseries for ourselves, no one else can help us. God cannot come down to help us. So we should learn to help ourselves. Everyone can do it, because human beings have free will. Each of us is fully equipped, each of us has all the resources, to create misery or happiness for ourselves.

In daily life, we use only a very small part of the mind—the conscious mind, that part which functions during the waking state. But what happens during the time we spend in dreaming and sleeping? To understand something about this, you might analyze your dreams, but this will not help you understand why you dream. It is more important to understand the dreaming state itself than it is to understand your dreams. What happens to you when you are in deep sleep? Why are you not attached to your belongings during that time? Why are you not aware of the person sleeping next to you, whom you love so much? Why do you completely withdraw and go into deep sleep? Nature is teaching you a lesson. It says, "It is good for you to love, but it is not good for you to be attached. That is why I am teaching you to withdraw yourself, though you are still with those objects while you sleep." To withdraw during sleep is a natural process that helps us to rest, but that rest is temporary; it does not give us complete solace, complete happiness, complete rest. There is not a single object in the world that can totally satisfy us. No experience in the waking, dreaming, or sleeping states can provide us with total bliss. When we analyze all the joys in the world, we realize that they all give only partial pleasure. Nothing gives eternal pleasure, yet people are in search of it, so they are actually students of eternal joy. The yogis say, "We receive only little joys from the world, but if we could expand these joys, they would become eternal joy." The momentary joys we experience in the world give us glimpses of higher joy. It is possible to attain that eternal joy.

The Three Selves

Human beings have three selves: the mortal self, the partially mortal self, and the immortal self. We should try to pay attention to all the moments of life and to attain that everlasting happiness here and now by understanding, by analyzing these three selves. The mortal self is that part which changes all the time. It includes the physical body and anything outside the body. There is nothing in this world that does not change, that does not decompose. Everything is subject to change, death, and decomposition. People search the earth for eternal joy, but they do not find it because the external world is temporary; it cannot give eternal joy. The body changes; it grows, and finally it decays. It is nothing but a minute drop in the ocean. The body falls apart and the conscious mind stops functioning when the two guards to the city of life stop doing their duty. When inhalation and exhalation stop, the body and mind cannot continue. So, the conscious mind, the breath, and the body are the mortal part of us.

When we leave this platform, the world, where do we go? Having left the world of action and the world of speech, we remain in our thinking world. After death we do not go to either hell or heaven; we remain in the atmosphere created by our own habits. If our habits are bad, we create hell for ourselves; but if we have created a good atmosphere by our actions and our thinking, then we are in heaven. There is no office somewhere in the clouds that keeps account of our deeds, but within us there is a wonderful, unique setup, the greatest of all computers, that records all our deeds and actions. This is called the unconscious mind. It is the account ledger of the past. The ledger is changed periodically, but not the accounting system.

The unconscious mind is like a vehicle that we are driving, and each of us is an individual because each of us has an individual vehicle. When we gain the power to release ourselves from the unconscious mind, then we are in the cosmos. The moment we get free from the vehicle, we are free forever. Each of us is an individual because each one has an individual unconscious mind that is different from others, and it is this which creates our individual personalities. When people die, they remain so closed within their individual thinking process—"I did this, I did that, I did not do this"—that they remain in individual consciousness all the time. This is the partially immortal self. The body, breath, and conscious mind are subject to change, death, and decomposition, but the individual soul is eternal. So where is the problem? The whole problem is with the mind; it creates a wall between you and the Reality. Through meditation, contemplation, and prayer, you can release yourself from individual boundaries and go to the totally immortal Self. The individual self is like a drop of water that expands and becomes the ocean, the cosmic Self. So qualitatively you and the Lord are one and the same, but quantitatively you are not; for that, you will have to make an effort. All these practices, all these rituals, that people do are just to train that magic-maker called the mind.

Turning Within

The human mind is bewildered, and it tries to find out where to find the answers to the questions of life. Some people search in the external world, but others seek within. These inner-directed people say that that which is in the cosmos is within, and that which is within is in the cosmos. So they go within to the source, to that point which is the universal cosmos. Those who are trying to research from the gross, to the grosser, and then to the grossest aspects of reality are called modern, or Western, philosophers. Those who try to go within and research in the interior world are called Eastern philosophers. Thus, the Eastern and Western concepts in philosophy have nothing to do with geographical boundaries. Eastern philosophers say that if you understand yourself, then you will understand the whole cosmos, and you will realize that the individual self is the Self of all. That is the greatest hope and joy that we receive. One's self is the Self of all: when you realize this, you can never hate anyone, because you realize that in hating someone you are hating yourself. Those who hate others are indulging in self-hatred; those who criticize others are criticizing themselves. They are not aware of that immortal, universal Self, which is the Self of all.

When you turn within, you understand that it is the mind that creates a barrier between you and the Reality. Many people who study meditation think that they should try to stop the mind from thinking, but this never happens. Many students think, "Oh, what a bad thought is coming. My method of meditation must not be good." The thought is not bad, but they become very caught up in it, and they allow those thought patterns to influence their body language. This does not allow them to be steady. The mind goes through fluctuations at a very high speed, and when you try to study the mind, you don't know how to handle it because no one has helped you train the mind.

What can help you train the mind? Nothing external can help. The yogis pray, "O Lord, let this external world not trouble me, so that I can go within." You should adjust your life so that the external world of objects and relationships does not disturb you when you are going within. The world can do only one great thing for students of meditation, and that is to not disturb them.

When you remove the obstacles that you have been creating, then you are enlightened. Enlightenment is not something that you gain; enlightenment is a state of mind that is free from pain and misery. Human beings can be analyzed by understanding all levels of life systematically. A human life can be compared to a lamp that is covered by progressively denser shades or sheaths. As you remove the dense outer coverings, you find more and more light, and finally a place full of light, with no darkness whatsoever. You are already enlightened, but you do not realize it because you are constantly identifying yourself with the outer sheaths and with the objects of the world. This is establishing a friendship with the weak, and that never helps. Friendship with the weak is dangerous, for you become dependent on those friends and expect too much, and then they say, "Sorry, we won't serve you, we cannot." The weak will leave you; when you leave the world they don't help you. They don't have that power; they decay. They are not good friends.

The Four Functions of Mind

On the path of the inner voice you should learn to adjust the external world so that it does not become a barrier to your interior research. But before you can really explore within, you must understand the four functions of mind. This diagram will help you see how they are coordinated:

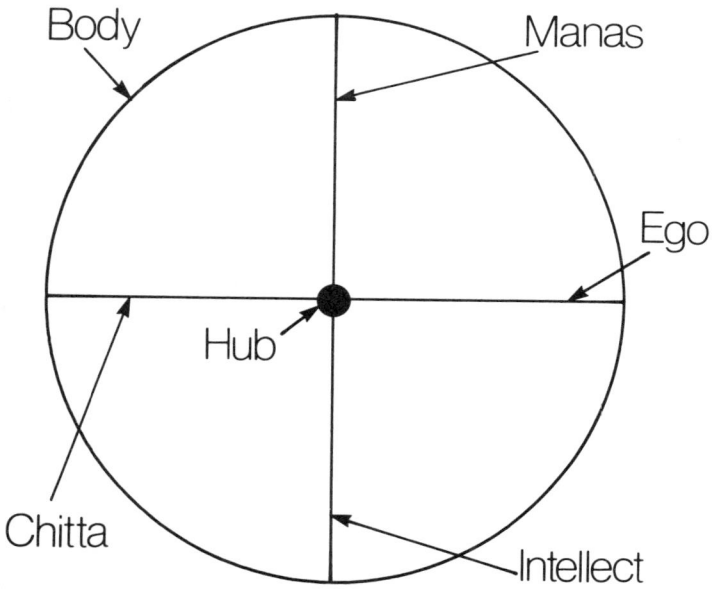

The body is like a wheel; it cannot rotate without its spokes. There are many spokes, but four of them are major: *manas*, ego, *buddhi*, and the storehouse, *chitta*. If you understand these spokes properly, you will understand the wheel as well. The spokes motivate the body to rotate, but they themselves are motivated to move by the hub. That center of consciousness within does not move, yet it makes everything go. It motivates all the functions of the body, and it motivates all the functions of the universe. That hub is called the individual soul.

Manas is a very powerful agent in the inner self. Whenever you have any doubt, it comes from manas. It helps the other faculties and gives account of them. If manas is weak, the whole interior self is disturbed. Manas functions both inside and out; it is like an importer and exporter. It has ten agents, called the senses, which help it know what is going on outside, what is going on inside, how to let things outside, and how to pull things inside. The word "manas" comes from the Sanskrit root *man*, which means "mind." The English word "man" also comes from this Sanskrit root, because the mind is that which makes you a man, a human being. That faculty of the mind which helps you identify with the body is the ego. You belong to light, but the ego says, "No, this is my body, this is me. That light is not me." The ego always identifies itself with external objects, forgetting the Reality. But there are two types of ego: the lower ego, which identifies with objects, and the higher ego, which can help you become aware of the Reality.

The *buddhi*, or intellect, is the faculty that decides, judges, and discriminates. When you think, "Shall I do it or not?" the intellect says, "Do it, you'll get this," or "Don't do it, it's not worth it." Like the ego, the intellect has two facets: higher and lower. The lower intellect works only with external matters and concerns and cannot go beyond this level. But the higher intellect comes in touch with the reservoir inside. When you purify the higher intellect, it can lead you to the infinite library of intuition within. Finally, the fourth function of the mind is *chitta*, the "mind-stuff." Chitta is the storehouse from which the flow of knowledge goes to all the various avenues and aspects of life.

When you understand the functions of the mind, you can establish inner coordination. But if you are not coordinated, you stumble, and inner stumbling creates a serious conflict for human beings. Inner conflict is the mother of all problems, because if there is conflict within, there will always be conflict without. How to be free from conflicts within and without is the only question in life. You shouldn't waste time in trying to know God—nothing of value will happen if you do this. Your duty is not to prove the existence of God but to make the mind aware of the Reality all the time. For this, you need to understand the mind so that it can be free from pain and conflict.

When the mind is calm, it does not create a wall between you and the Reality, and you can then see the Reality face to face. That is called God. God is the center of power, life, light, and love. By having inner strength, by having inner control, by loving, you can do tremendous good for others. Many times, through foolishness, ignorance, and lack of training, you might hurt others, but you can constantly make the effort to calm the mind so you are aware of the Reality all the time. When the lake of life is calm, you can see what is at the bottom of the lake. Then the individual self realizes the cosmic Self, the Self of all. That is why you do meditation, contemplation, or prayer. All inner paths are valid, but on the external path you can be misguided, you can have accidents. On the inner path, you will always get help from the center of truth, for the quest of truth is always helpful. We are all children of truth and immortality and eternity. But before you can understand and realize this, you must learn to analyze yourself.

Selfless Service: Pathway to Freedom

Seventh International Congress, New York City, June 20, 1982

We all talk about freedom, but before we can be free from misery we must come to understand the nature and source of our suffering. Whether you are an atheist or a believer in God, you will have to agree that no human being can live without doing actions. And whether you are a religionist, a philosopher, or a scientist, you will have to accept one law: As you sow, so shall you reap. All human beings have to perform actions, and then reap the fruits of those actions. But the fruits motivate them to do more actions, and thus a chain reaction occurs. In this way people create a whirlpool for themselves and then become trapped in it. Then they go to temples, churches, and synagogues, to pandits, swamis, and priests in an effort to get freedom from their miseries. But my conviction is that we alone can liberate ourselves from our miseries because we alone have created them; no one else has created any misery for you. Self-created misery is responsible for your bondage, and you alone can free yourself from that misery.

The only way to do this liberation is through selfless service performed skillfully and lovingly. To be selfless is a great joy. Exactly as someone develops a love for classical music, you can also create a love for being selfless. As you gradually come to learn the lessons of daily life, you begin to realize that human resources should not be wasted on self-gratification alone. The understanding slowly dawns that the suffering we see all over the world is due to the ignorance called selfishness and that selfless action alone can help humanity.

123

Some people talk of the path of renunciation, and others talk about the path of action, but actually we simply need to learn how to live in the world, yet remain above—like a lotus that grows in the mud and water and yet remains unaffected by them. How does one live in the world and yet remain unaffected? We cannot live without performing actions, and we are bound to receive the fruits of those actions. So that which binds you is not your duties, but the fruits that you receive. When you learn to offer those fruits to the people with whom you live, you will be doing your duties, and yet you will be free.

Modern culture has polluted our civilization so much that it shocks us when someone does something without a selfish motive. We cannot accept it; we cannot assimilate the idea that someone would do something for us and ask for nothing in return. When I left the Himalayas, I came to Detroit to attend a conference, and whenever I did something for someone, they would ask, "Why are you doing this for me? What do you want from me?" If it was a woman, she thought that I had a questionable motive; if it was a man, he thought that I was after his money. For several months I did not know why people were reacting like this, but slowly I realized that I was not acting the way people act in the modern world. I found that if you do something without any selfishness, people will misunderstand you, and that when you are surrounded by selfish people, your positive qualities will be abused.

Home Education

The art of living and being is not taught in our schools or homes. The seeds sown in childhood are stronger than the seeds sown in adulthood. Most problems come from defects in childhood training, and the main center where children receive training is the home. Therefore the family institution needs to be completely transformed; for if the home life is not properly organized, then it is not able to impart proper education, and without proper education we will never be able to create a new society.

A transformation of society can be brought about only by

introducing real education at home. If this is done, many of the major problems of today—such as hatred, jealousy, and self-ishness—will disappear. The basic education for wise parents to impart to their children is practical education: how to enjoy giving, how to enjoy serving others, how to enjoy being still. It is very difficult to close your eyes and meditate if you have not been trained in childhood. You may close your eyes and imitate your meditation teacher, but nothing happens if the mind remains preoccupied. Proper training in childhood is a necessity. If parents teach their children at an early age to give and to find joy in giving, they will never be sad. If you start practicing these precepts now at home, then your children will learn these qualities, and the future generation will be happy.

Improvement is impossible without practice. And today practical Christianity, Judaism, and Hinduism are missing in the world: they are not being practiced. We have sufficient religions—we know what to do and what not to do—but people do not know how to be because they do not apply practical methods of spirituality in their lives. But once they begin to receive that education which is needed in childhood—and so learn to give, to serve, and to enjoy serving—then they will enjoy mental and spiritual health. In today's society no one teaches children how to give, and so they never learn how to love; and if someone does not learn how to love, how can they maintain a healthy relationship? It is not possible to separate life from relationship. They are one and the same thing—two sides of the same coin. As long as we live, we will have relationships. Even if we renounce the world, we cannot run away from the concept of relationship because the body, breath, and mind are related to the spirit. We are related to people where we work, to people with whom we live. People aspire to be happy with their spouse and children, and yet they are not happy because they are selfish. No relationship in the world can be happy if one is selfish. Relationships are considered to be very important these days, but they are not harmonious because everyone is selfish. Everyone is unhappy, and the more selfish we are, the more unhappy we are. If the wife learns to give to the husband, and the husband learns to give to the wife, then there will be great harmony and happiness. But if they expect too much from each other, there will be no harmony; there will only be expectation, and expectation is the mother of all miseries.

Prayer Means Selfless Service

The misery that you are experiencing is self-created; there is no God, no principle of nature, that creates misery for you. God, the law of equality, will never make anyone miserable and will never make anyone happy. As long as your expectations are fulfilled, you think that you are happy, but you are only deceiving yourself and killing your conscience. You repeatedly murder yourself, and yet you think that by going to church you will find happiness. But no God can ever come down and free you from your self-created misery. Prayer cannot liberate you, prayer can inspire you, but in practical life, selfless service alone is the real prayer that gives you freedom from the bondage that you constantly create for yourself. It also gives freedom to others, for you become an example. Performing your duties consciously and renouncing the fruits of your actions for the sake of selfless service is the greatest of all worships. But worshiping in a church, worshiping a statue, or worshiping your teacher does not help much.

There is a story that demonstrates this nicely. There were two gardeners in a rich man's garden, and both were very honest and loving. Whenever the rich man visited the garden, one of the gardeners always adored him like a lord. "O master, you look so handsome! You are a beautiful, wonderful man; I love you. When you come I cannot do any work, but I just want to look at you. I constantly remember you. I want to be with you all the time." The other gardener remained silent. He would continue to do his duties conscientiously, and in the evening he would bring all the fruits of his actions to his master. So one gardener worked for his master, and the other flattered him all the time.

People do the same thing when they pray—"O God, you are great." God already knows that he is great. Such prayers do not help in self-unfoldment and self-enlightenment. What can prayers do? What can the Bible do? It is good to respect all the great Bibles and religious founders of the world, but that respect, that mere reverence, does not transform the personality. In my own life, for many years I often went to the temple and recited many prayers, but when I came out of the temple I always found that my habits were the same as before. Nothing happened to me; my prayers did not change me. For there is a law, accepted by all the great Bibles and philosophies of the world, that states that we have to reap the fruits of our actions. No matter how many times we pray, this law is not going to be altered. We can pray the whole day—and doing so may inspire us or give us some solace—but our personality will not be transformed. For thousands of years people have been going to temples and worshiping their personal gods, but that has not transformed either them or their society. You can shackle yourself a hundred times to the wall of a church, but this is not going to help you. What will help you is learning to offer the fruits of your actions joyfully, selflessly, and skillfully. Then you will find yourself free, really free, all the time.

Transformation of personality can take place only when you accept the responsibility of understanding your own character. When you begin to examine your character, you see that it is made of nothing but habit patterns. Actions repeated many times form a habit; a groove is created, and the mind begins to flow spontaneously to that groove. If habit patterns are not changed, you cannot change your character, and thus you cannot transform your personality. Many habits are so deep-rooted that you do not understand them, and even though you pray, study, and practice, it is all in vain—nothing happens. Most deep-rooted habits are formed in childhood, and the so-called education imparted in the schools and universities is not helpful in learning how to deal with them and change them. But you can learn to modify your behavior by realizing that it has three aspects that can be trained: mind, action, and speech. Even if you do not understand much about the mind, you can analyze your actions and speech. If you just learn to be aware of what you are saying and doing, you will realize how much energy you waste by misusing your speech and action. But if you learn to use your speech and action selflessly to serve others, you will find that they become very powerful.

Motivations for Giving

Selfless service is not to be done only for the sake of others, only to please others. It should be done because it liberates you, because it makes you happy. It is a great joy—the highest of all joys in the world. Selfless service is more helpful to the person who performs it than to the person for whom it is performed. Not all service is selfless: people are charitable for three reasons. Some people give to charity so their name will be known all over and thus their business will flourish because others will think that they are very good—not only rich but generous. Other people give, thinking that if they give now, they will receive in the next world. But very few people give with the knowledge that holding onto anything only creates problems and so they should offer all they have in order to be free. This third kind of charity gives freedom, but the first two only create more bondage. The actions are the same, but the motivations are different.

If you do an action that is not helpful to you, it will give you fruits that are not helpful. When you understand this, you will realize that selfless service is the highest of all worships. No prayer can be compared with such action. Yet merely realizing this truth intellectually is not enough. Many people understand this truth, yet they do not worship through selfless service. We must practice this truth in our lives. In doing this, we should constantly be aware of the fact that other human beings are like shrines, and that the inner dweller in each of us is God. Thus by serving others we serve God. When we understand this, then instead of building temples, churches, and mosques, we can use our time, energy, and money to help others in practical ways. Selfless service is the finest of all prayers, and we need this sort of prayer in the world. Thinking that God is in a building and then running there to worship makes the human mind dependent; then you lose self-confidence and never realize that you are someone special or that there is something divine within you. The Bible says that a human being is a living temple of the Holy Spirit, and you should remain constantly aware of this fact.

No matter how much we pray, there is only one ray of hope for our generation and the next generation, and that is to learn how to enjoy selfless service. For ages, humanity has been trying to attain the next step in its evolvement, but it has not yet attained it because people are becoming more, not less, self-centered. We are therefore creating more miseries for ourselves. People listen to lectures, study books, and say they will practice, but what is there to be practiced? You should simply understand the truth and then follow it. What good will meditation do if for five or ten minutes in the morning you become a sage and then the rest of the day you are a monster? That kind of practice is never going to help you. Meditation is conscious action, and meditation in action is very important. If you do meditation in action, then wherever you are, you will remain aware of the center of consciousness within, and you will be in samadhi the whole day. Your whole life will be a lovely poem and a beautiful song. Only meditation in action can help the flower of humanity to bloom.

This is something very realistic to be practiced if you really want to improve, if you want to unfold, if you want to enlighten yourself. Attaining enlightenment does not mean receiving or achieving something; enlightenment is the absence of bondage. When you are free from all miseries, then you gain freedom, and that state which is free from pains and miseries is called enlightenment. You have all the potentials, powers, and resources to free yourself from the bondages you have created for yourself. If you do not know how to do this, if you feel lost and think that you have committed many mistakes, then just start practicing selfless service. The simplest way to be selfless is to learn to serve the people with whom you live. This is the greatest of all prayers.

Humanity is suffering because we have forgotten one simple principle. Why are my hands and feet working? Ultimately for my mouth. Why do my mouth and teeth chew my food? For my liver. Why is my liver functioning? For my whole being. In the same way, each person should function for the whole of humanity. But instead, people are interested only in themselves, and this selfishness makes them miserable. Instead of creating this misery, we can create happiness in the world by serving others according to our capacity. Selfless service alone is the way to freedom. We do not need any other formula than that.

Articles

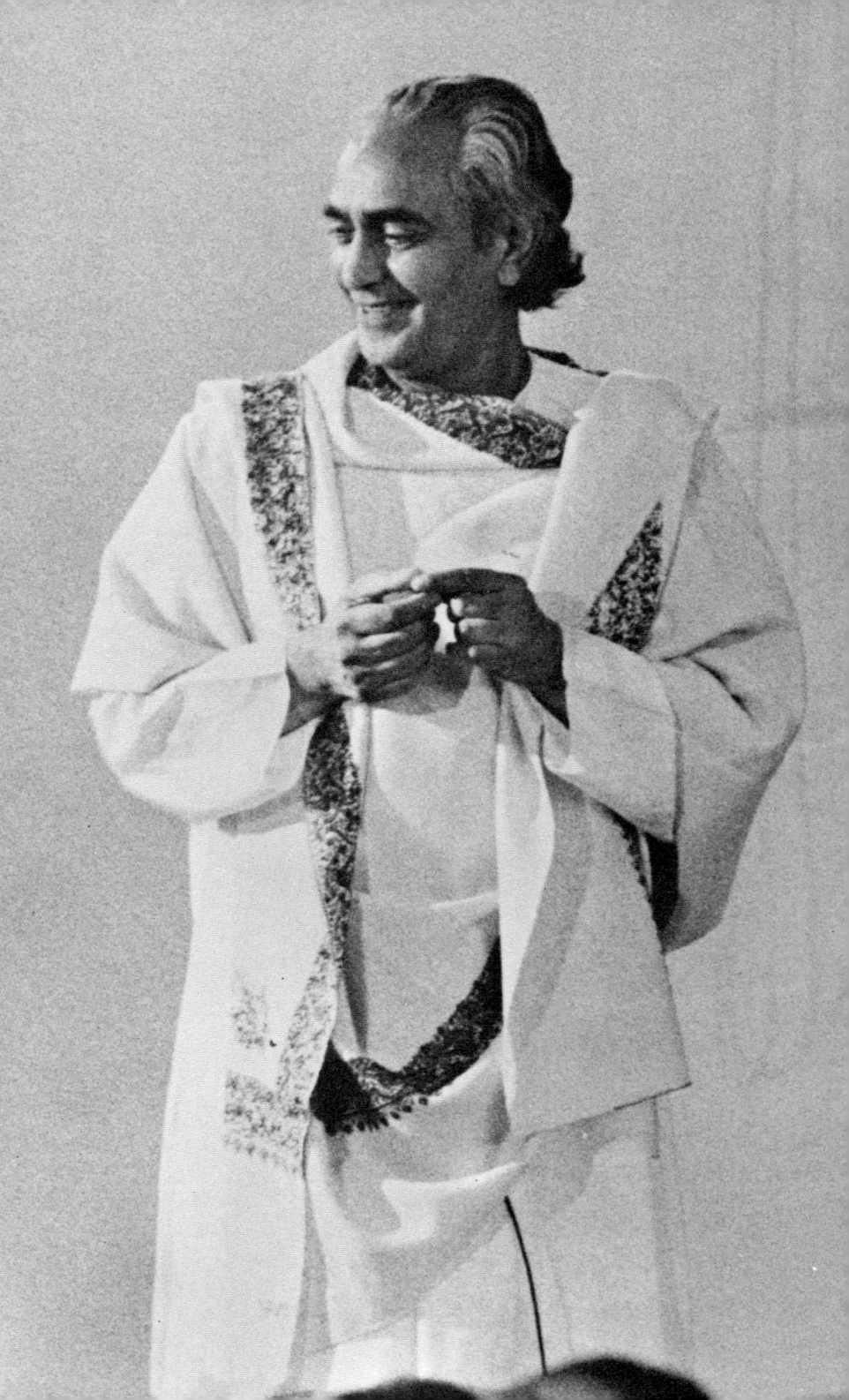

Religion and Modern Humanity

From Voice of the Himalayas, *Vol. 2, no. 2 (Fall, 1972)*

Can religion inspire the modern person? Can religion give any positive solution to the situations of today? Can it solve the problems of modern people? We are living in an age of materialism. Wealth tempts people like a deceptive mirage. It hardens the heart and causes pride, making us forget our own real self. The materialistic civilization of our age has made the modern person an instrument who is being played in the hands of insincerity and untruthfulness. The rudderless ship of human civilization is heading toward the rocks of hatred, aimless living, and eventual self-destruction. The present world is full of fear, suspicion, quarrels, and struggles. The philosophy of flesh substitutes license for discipline and self-indulgence for self-sacrifice. The ideal of religion is forgotten and lost; only a poor external structure remains.

Scientists have conquered the air and the atom, but, alas, people have not realized the mysteries of the real Self, the *Atman*. We have journeyed to the moon and explored outer space, but we have not conquered our archenemy, the mind. A person is a soul wearing a physical body, and the soul is extremely subtle; it is beyond the realm of physical science. Material science knows nothing of thought, of the origin of life, or of the destiny of human nature and the universe. Religion alone can give the answers to such questions. Actually, religion is the most rational science, the science of life itself, the science of humankind as it essentially is.

The real basis of all science is Yoga Vedanta science. Modern science is based on observations and senses, but sensing is false knowledge. Science analyzes and classifies phenomena, while the Yoga Vedanta scientific religion teaches one to transcend phenomena and attain immortality. Religion is intuitive knowledge. It is not a matter of belonging to any particular caste, creed, sex, or color; rather, it is a matter of evolving deeper insight and understanding and expressing these through life.

Religion is life. It is realization and becoming. Religion is a living experience in the life of a person. Real religion is the religion of the heart, but the heart must be purified first. Religion is a manifestation of the eternal glow of the Self within us, and the main purpose of religion is the unfoldment of this inner divinity. A life of selfless service and sacrifice, with regular efforts for realization and meditation, are the chief pillars of religion. This is the highest religion, for the practice of religion is the practice of goodness, justice, truth, love, and purity.

The singing notes of true religion are "Be good, do good, be pure, be kind, serve all, love all, and exclude none." The practice of these precepts alone will awaken people to consciousness of the unity of existence and realization of the divinity within and without. Selfless service purifies the heart and opens it for the receipt of divine light. So, cheer up a person who is in distress, encourage a person who is in despair, and remove sorrow by your kind and loving words. Smile and make another person smile. Be a lamp to those who have lost their way. Be a boat and a bridge to those who want to reach the other shore, the shore of fearlessness and happiness. Do your duty to the best of your ability, and leave the rest to God. All your actions should be with detachment and for all, in the spirit of dedication to the divine. Then your actions will not bind you. Vedanta says, "Ye friends, spiritualize all your activities. Be kind; speak with sweetness; be thou as truthful, brave, pure, and loving as Buddha, Krishna, Christ, and Muhammad."

Those who feed their minds with thoughts of God, their hearts with purity, and their hands with selfless service are truly religious. Concerning such people Vedanta says, "Then where is bondage, where is sorrow, when the unity in diversity is realized?" God has a master plan, and we all have our parts to play. Play out your part well. Realize your Self, and you will swim in the ocean of divine bliss and happiness. As long as there is the least identification with the body and selfishness, one cannot expect Self-realization. All pleasure and pain, gain and loss, are mental creations. Thou art the immortal Self! It is the physical body, the lower self, that goes and comes.

Real Religion Is One

Look within, try to remove your defects—this is practical Vedanta religion. Visiting temples, churches, or mosques regularly and learning prayers or mantras by heart is easy, but the removal of defects requires a great deal of struggle for many years. Religion begins where the intellect ends. An impure heart cannot understand or enjoy religion; it cannot realize the Reality. The fundamental principles of all religions are equally good, if they are brought into practice. All the sacred books of the East and West are full of formulas, precepts, and commandments. Why then do the various religions not satisfy the questions of modern seekers? Why do they not solve the problems of modern people? Because the leaders of religion today do not try to bring down the mighty ideals of their religions into practice for the common person. Their approach is not scientific. But religion itself is actually a pure science, the science of life. Religion is practical philosophy, and philosophy is theoretical religion. Philosophy is forever searching, inquiring, questioning, and sensing, but religion is a scientific process that brings philosophy into practice. Religion is realizing and experiencing in the true sense.

Religion is one because God is one; but many are the forms of practice and expression. The same type of jacket cannot suit all people. Individual temperaments and traditional, historical, and geographical backgrounds differ—hence the need for different religions. All the religions exist to enlighten their people in all the spheres of life. One religion is as good as another; one path to the

Supreme is as good as any other path. Cows have different colors, but the color of milk is always the same. Similarly, although there are many religious sects, God is one. So in essence there can be only one religion, although in practice it has many forms. Diversity is the order and law of creation, and religious practice is no exception to this universal rule.

What is needed today is for people to come out truthfully, crossing the sectarian barriers that separate them and breaking the chains of fanaticism and dogmatism. Then alone can religion serve the purpose of modern humanity. Let not personal bias, force, conventions, or the opinions of fanatics and sectarians blind your vision into a narrow view of religion. One must be able to differentiate the essential from the nonessential in religion and philosophy through the power of pure reason and discrimination. The essentials of all religions are one and the same; religions differ only in the nonessentials. According to yoga science, religion is the most rational science. It is the science of life itself, the science of humankind as it essentially is, not merely as it is presumed to be.

Real religion is one, and it is the religion of realization of truth and love. Truth is neither Hindu nor Muhammedan, neither Buddhist nor Christian. Truth is one homogeneous, eternal substance. Truth alone can liberate humanity. Many preach Buddhism, but still no one gives up desires and violence. Many preach Christianity, but no one practices love. Many preach Islam, but no one recognizes the universal brotherhood. So is the case with Hinduism also: no one realizes the divinity in all. The preaching of religion has become a livelihood, while the actual practice of religion has become an object of scorn. Therefore, let everyone practice his or her own religion and strive to attain the goal. Let religion create saints and yogis rather than temples, mosques, and churches. Let modern humanity believe in itself. It does not matter whether one believes in God or not. Believing in "self" is believing in God. So, there is no room for nonbelieving in God, because we all believe in our own self-existence.

All religions have their founders. Whenever any important truth has been suppressed by the arrogance and selfishness of a priestly class for its own selfish ends, there has appeared a great saint or prophet to emphasize the truth, to remove the dross concealing it, and to make it shine in its original brilliance, purity, splendor, and glory. Real religion is one; it is the religion of truth and love; it is the religion of the heart; it is the religion of selfless service, goodness, kindness, and tolerance.

The Religion of Knowledge and Love

I belong to that religion which is extremely catholic and liberal and which pays respect to all religions. I am a Bharati, and my country is Bharat. *Bha* and *rat* mean "knowledge" and "love." My Vedanta religion is the religion of love and knowledge. The words *Bharat* and *Bharati* are mentioned several times in the Vedas, the oldest books in the library of humanity. Vedanta philosophy is the ultimate source of my religion, and this philosophy reveals the most subtle spiritual truths. Even Western scholars have paid tribute to the seers of Vedanta. Vedanta was not founded by any single prophet. The seers of knowledge founded Vedanta, and anyone who practices Yoga Vedanta can become a seer. The teachings of the *rishis* (seers) of yore do not pertain to Hindus alone, for they are of an all-embracing universal nature. They are meant for the people of the whole world. The Bhagavad Gita and the Upanishads teach universal religion, but fanatics have given them a sectarian coloring. What a pity!

One who follows the path of absolute Truth is a saint, and saints are never sectarian. They are for the people of the world; nowhere have I found that they were only for the Hindus, or for any other particular group. I am proud to call myself a Bharati and to state that my religion is Vedanta, which is universal. Vedanta gives a complete view of life. It is free from fanaticism, and it has various thoughts on philosophy. It is more a league of religions than a single religion with a definite creed. It is the fellowship of faith. It prescribes spiritual food and provides for good conduct in life for one and all according to each individual's qualifications and growth. It loves all and excludes none.

If any group in society performs its functions and duties

honestly, sincerely, and selflessly with full devotion, I call that being religious. If science, art, technology, or any other field contribute something to humanity's progress, I think that they are following religion in its true sense. But all this progress should have as its aim the welfare of humanity. We suffer on account of our selfishness, so religion asks all fields of endeavor not to exhibit selfishness but to work on the problems of progress selflessly. Thus true religion is progressive; it is not a barrier in any sphere of life. It is purely scientific, and it should be accepted by all—here, there, and everywhere. True religion has been progressive from the very beginning of the history of humankind and is still progressive today, if rightly understood and practiced. This one true religion of humankind is not to be confused with the pseudo-concept of religion, which has been responsible for so much bloodshed in human history.

If the codes of Vedanta are tested in the laboratory of any human life, they will always give positive results. Vedanta says to you, "All this belongs to God because God has been manifested in all the names and forms of this world. All the things are for you; enjoy them. But remember, they are not yours. Do not exploit anyone's rights. Work for God, and be detached. Live a long life working selflessly for the sake of all beings, because God is in all." Thus you are free when you follow and practice religion.

Vedanta is a synthesis of all the types of religious experience. If religion is practiced, it can enlighten individuals, nations, and humankind at large. In this way human society can progress in all directions and on all levels. Even in the rush and roar of modern civilization, in the busy cities of this world, an individual can be elevated and benefited by the practice of religion. Through the practice of religion we can make the better society for which we all aspire; we can help the human race and save the world from degeneration and disaster.

What Is Yoga?

From the All-India Yoga Conference Brochure, October 27-29, 1973

Yoga is a Sanskrit word derived from the root word *yug*, which means "to join." In yoga the embodied spirit, or the individual Self (*Atman*), is united with the supreme universal Self (*Paramatman*). The methods of the various schools of yoga differ, but the goal is one. This practice is an exact science. Patanjali, the codifier of this science, describes yoga as the control of thought. Here "thought" is not used in the narrow sense of reflection, but should be taken to include sense perception, imagination, and dreams.

Yoga has also been defined as the science that raises the capacity of the human mind to perceive, assimilate, and respond to the infinite Consciousness, from which all aspects of the universe are created. In fact, yoga makes the aspirant a transmitting as well as a receiving agent of such infinite, subtle activities. It then becomes easy to receive the unspoken thoughts of others from any distance. It also becomes easy to communicate one's own thoughts in order to assist others in spiritual upliftment and to guide them in difficulties. By means of this science, saints and sages of all times have performed many deeds generally referred to as miracles. The same tradition is being carried on by their followers even today, although there are only a fortunate few of them.

Among all the sciences of the world, yoga science is the highest. This science has two parts—theoretical and practical. The theory can be learned through scriptures and books, but without a perfect guru, the practical part is impossible. So a student of yoga should be careful in choosing a guru. How does one know who is a true yogi? This is a serious problem these days because modern society does not make sincere inquiries and is therefore generally swindled by imposters. A true yogi will always encourage his disciple to practice yoga systematically; a real yogi will never misguide or mislead. A true yogi is one who has reached the final state of samadhi or bliss.

There are various yoga disciplines, and all of them lead to final freedom and perfection. Those who dedicate the fruits of their deeds to God are called Karma yogis. There is another school known as Bhakti yoga that believes in the absolute surrender of all desires, and even one's self, to God. This particular school does not aspire to immediate liberation; it is the path of devotion. The third school is Jnana yoga, the highest of the yogas. In it the soul is recognized as identical with the absolute Reality. Other yogas are Hatha yoga, Mantra yoga, Laya yoga, and Kundalini yoga. The word "yoga" when used in a restricted sense refers to the *Ashtanga* (eightfold) yoga of Patanjali, which is also called Raja yoga. Yoga science depends on the basic code given by the yogi gurus who have attained superconscious knowledge. This tradition leads to the highest state of samadhi (the blissful state), and it has developed certain principles and disciplines so that the young yogi may follow the path more easily. Raja yoga is a royal road on which the milestones are fixed, and when it is trodden properly, the road continues to guide the student.

According to Patanjali, the eight steps of Raja yoga are *yama, niyama, asana, pranayama, pratyahara, dharana, dhyana,* and *samadhi.* The first two parts, yama and niyama, contain the ten commitments of yoga. Without practicing these disciplines, the aspirant should not expect any progress. The third part is posture, the fourth is breathing, and the fifth is control of the senses. These five are the external parts. The last three are concentration, meditation, and the superconscious state. These are the internal parts of the eightfold practice of yoga.

The first four rungs of the yoga ladder are Hatha yoga practices. Hatha yoga concerns physical culture and breath control, but Raja yoga deals with the mind and its modifications. Raja yoga and Hatha yoga are interdependent; they are necessary counterparts of each other. No one can become a perfect yogi without knowledge and practice of both parts. Raja yoga begins where properly practiced Hatha yoga ends. The spiritual path is as sharp as the edge of a razor. Aspirants with strong determination, undaunted spirit, and indomitable courage successfully tread this path in a short period. When one definitely makes up one's mind to tread this path, everything becomes smooth and easy. There is a descent of grace from the Lord, and the aspirant is aided by vibrations from the spiritual world.

The fifth step is control of the senses. When the mind is stilled through the evenness of the breath, or through the word given by the teacher, or through sound vibrations, the aspirant controls the senses. Controlling the senses means being always aware of the sense organs and learning to direct them properly.

The sixth step is concentration. A Raja yogi starts his practice with the mind and acquires *siddhis* (special powers) by the practice of concentration and meditation. In concentration the dissipated powers of the mind are gathered together and directed toward one object by means of voluntary attention. Voluntary attention is developed through perseverance. As interest develops attention, so attention develops interest. Concentration is possible only when the practice of voluntary attention is strengthened. Voluntary attention and its application is a wonderful tool in both the material and spiritual worlds.

It is through meditation alone that a person can reach the superconscious (blissful) state; through meditation alone the hidden treasures deeply buried in the subconscious mind are brought under a state of harmonious control. Most diseases have their origin at the subconscious level, and without meditation it is not possible to reach this level of consciousness. Therefore it is necessary to introduce meditation to everyone, so that all may be made capable of analyzing and utilizing the vital hidden portion of their minds. Human beings are unaware of the latent power within themselves. Without meditation a person cannot reach the subtler realms. During meditation one comes face to face with problems and deals with them properly. If humanity is to achieve a better civilization, it has to nurture the growth of the inner being, which develops from the direct and continued experience of proper meditation.

Deepest meditation, or samadhi, is the final rung of the Raja yoga ladder. One who has achieved this state is blessed, for he has perfect control over his mind and actions. In this state a person becomes one with the Divine Self. This is the state that can be classified as sleepless sleep, a state of union and permanent bliss.

Yoga is not a religion. It is a scientific approach to life. Religion tells one what to do, but yoga teaches one how to be. Yoga is a divine science that furnishes the means to educate and develop the whole person. The whole process of yoga is an ascent into the purity of the absolute perfection that is the original state of humankind. Yoga science is the soul of all the sciences and philosophies, and it can solve the basic problems of modern humanity everywhere.

Beginning the Practice of Meditation

Compiled from lectures for Dawn, *Vol. 3, no. 4 (Fall, 1983)*

The method of meditation is an inward process that finally leads one to the fountain of life and light. This is the center of consciousness, from where consciousness flows on various degrees and grades. A human being is a citizen of two worlds: the world within and the world without. To create a bridge between these two requires human effort, but it is possible for one to do so; it is possible to live in the world and yet remain above it. This art of living and being has its source in the method of meditation. That which cannot be taught by modern education can be understood and realized by practicing meditation. No one teaches modern people how to be still, and they never find the time and opportunity to be still. To be still is a must for meditation; for only then can the truth or the Reality within reveal itself. So meditation is a method of knowing truth, that which is within every human being. Meditating is a small technique that can be learned in a few minutes, but it is a very practical subject, and the benefits of meditation are immense.

There are many steps for attaining the highest state of meditation, and anyone who desires to practice can attain a state of meditation within a few months. The first benefit of meditation is freedom from stress and strain; the second benefit is clarity of mind; the third benefit is knowledge of one's own internal states. Then one is etablished in one's essential nature, which is happiness, peace, and bliss. Meditation helps one to attain the highest level of equilibrium and tranquility. With persistence, it leads one to the state of *turiya*, the state beyond.

But to attain these benefits, one must understand that knowledge is within and that one will have to practice. Practice will make one perfect. Without practice, one cannot have experience, and without experience one cannot be guided. Experience should be one's guide. This requires that one learn to discipline oneself. Discipline does not mean that someone should impose discipline on someone else; it means that one should learn to discipline oneself. In American life, in this affluent society, people do not understand the value of discipline. They think discipline is something very bad, that it is being told what not to do. Even parents do not discipline their children—because they themselves are not disciplined. They don't impart any exemplary education, environmental education, home education; so education is received from the colleges and universities, and that is not sufficient.

That which one learns from the so-called education that is imparted all over the world is mere information. People do not realize anything; they only receive information—what to do and what not to do. No one tells them how to be. Real education starts when one starts educating oneself. Whatever one has learned, that learning should go through inner filtration. How can one apply the education that one has received? Human beings have tremendous potentials; they can do wonders. History shows how a human being can lead masses and sacrifice himself for the masses, how he can become a symbol of selflessness. Discipline makes one aware of how to become selfless.

An Inward Method

As long as a person remains a petty individual, arrested by body consciousness, he will not enjoy life because he is still selfish, and whatever he does, he does for selfish motives. Real enjoyment comes when one starts renouncing for others: "I do not need it; I do not want it. Come on, you have it; you enjoy it." In a relationship, that selflessness is very important. But relationships in modern society are crumbling because every individual is becoming more selfish. People do not understand the law of truth or unfoldment. That law is called expansion, and meditation is the method for expanding one's consciousness.

Most people are not satisfied as they are, and so they are still seeking, but they are afraid of searching. And even if they are not afraid, still they do not know how to seek or where to seek, within or without. People are accustomed to searching in the external world because they have been taught to examine things, to verify things, in the external world. But nobody teaches them how to see within, how to look within, how to think, how to come to certain conclusions, how to decide, and how to take action according to their own decisions. All individuals should know themselves from within and without both. There are many means furnished by our society, by our educational system, to study and understand the external world, but there is no concrete education that gives people the means to watch within, to verify within.

Meditation shows one how to learn to know within oneself. There is no mystery in this method. It is a practical and systematic technique that leads one to peace and knowledge. If one knows all the things of the world and does not realize one's inner potentials, how can one enjoy life, and how can one attain the purpose of life? The greatest of all enjoyments is the tranquil state that can be attained through meditation. So often students get excited and want to attain the highest state in a few days' time, forgetting that this inward method is not like other learning programs. It is an unlearning program, a journey without movement—one advances without any movement. One remains still and yet attains one's goal.

Meditation Is Not Religion

Meditation teaches one how to be; it is an inward method for knowing oneself on all levels and for experiencing the higher levels of consciousness. The basic instruction for meditation is "Be still and know that I am God," and this is also the very core of the Bible. But meditation does not interfere with any religious or cultural beliefs. Meditation should not be mingled with any sort of religion, and religious ceremony should not be involved in meditation. Doing so could create needless conflict with one's cultural and religious background and personal beliefs. If a teacher involves any religious ceremony in meditation, it would be better not to learn from that person.

The word "meditation" has been used by various religions, but not with its proper meaning; real meditation is entirely different from the sense in which the word is used by religionists. The different religious groups of the world give people a code for what to do and what not to do, but the question of how to be remains unanswered. In the English dictionary the word "meditation" has not been explained as yet. It is defined as meaning to ruminate on, to reflect upon, to contemplate—that's all. But in the Sanskrit, Tibetan, Chinese, and Japanese languages, the word "meditation" has been used in a very clear way: it means to make the mind free from disturbing thoughts. Meditation is a method that makes one aware of the Reality. This is an inward journey from the gross, to the subtle, to the most subtle aspect of one's being.

The purpose of the school of meditation is to lead one to the center of consciousness, from where consciousness flows on various degrees and grades. The purpose of meditation is not to convert one from Christianity, for example, to Judaism, or from Hinduism to Zen. Meditation neither rejects nor recognizes any particular religion. The school of meditation is an inward method that leads one to the center of consciousness by stilling the mind. There is no other way of education that helps one to know oneself on all levels. There is no religion that does this, either—and if there is any philosophy that speaks of this, it is not helpful, because it is purely theoretical without any practice.

The practical aspect of religion is missing from daily life, no matter which religious tradition one comes from. "Knowing thyself" is the aim of everyone's life, and for that, one must practice an inward method. The ancients of all great religions of the world knew the method of meditation, but modern humanity is lost in the charms and attractions of materialism. This is a self-created misery. People are supposed to become wiser with age, but today old people are sent to state hospitals. Why does this happen? Because they are not taught to practice meditation and cannot deal with the loneliness of old age. People do not learn how to control their emotions. When Christ was on the cross, why did he not cry? The reply that he was suffering for us is not a sufficient answer. The answer is that there is a center within every human being that, if attained, gives freedom from all pains, fears, and miseries—even the fear of death evaporates. Christ attained that level; why then don't all Christians attain that state today? Because the great meditative practices of ancient Christianity have been lost. Practical Christianity does not exist today. If one really studies and understands the Scriptures, one wonders how the sages lived on Mount Athos. How did the Desert Fathers live? Could they live without meditation? It is not possible. A man who does not know meditation can go insane if he lives all alone.

What Meditation Isn't

Just as many people think meditation is a part of religion, they also confuse the words "meditation" and "contemplation." If one looks up the word "meditation" in the dictionary, he will find it defined as "contemplation," and "contemplation" is defined as "meditation," as if there were no difference between the two. But they are actually two different things. Thinking with a definite idea in mind is contemplation, but in meditation one does not explore the various aspects of a particular concept. In meditation one has decided on a single point of focus, and one does not change that—it is always the same focus. For contemplation one needs an idea, but to learn meditation one needs an object of concentration.

Meditation will tell one how distracted one's mind is, how much concentration one has, but meditation is different from concentration. To concentrate is to narrow down, to lead the mind one-pointedly in one direction. Meditation is expansion, but if the mind is scattered and dissipated, there is nothing to expand. Without concentration, meditation is not possible. Some schools of meditation want to please people, and so they say that one does not have to do anything particular to practice meditation. But they are cheating and hurting the people because it is not possible to direct the mind inward one-pointedly without concentration.

Meditation is a self-reliant method of inner study, and it therefore should not be confused with anything like hypnosis. Hypnosis can definitely help one in dealing with many dissipated and distorted conditions of the mind, and a therapist should use all the available resources to help the patient to find out something new, creative, and helpful. Sometimes hypnosis should be used, so I'm not going to reject it. But it does not make one independent, and so it cannot be included in a self-training program. Auto-suggestion cannot be part of a self-training program either. I used to practice hypnosis, and I have made experiments with it, but I do not pursue it anymore because it can be dangerous. In the unconscious there lie many, many levels, and sometimes one can lose touch with the person he has hypnotized. The person can go beyond the subconscious, and it is such a pleasurable state that he might refuse to come back. Freud also realized this problem. After he used this method, he found out that the patient can sometimes come in touch with certain powers within—negative or positive—that are beyond the reach of the therapist. I know a psychiatrist who used hypnosis for many years, who is now a patient herself because of overdoing it. Modern education is totally based on hypnosis, on suggestion. Education based on suggestion and autosuggestion is superficial and is not truthful.

What is the difference between hypnosis and meditation? Many of the books written on this topic are by people who have not experienced both systems, and so they cannot understand the differences between them. Hypnosis controls the mind, and then one is not oneself, but meditation is beneath all these different forms and names. The purpose of the school of meditation is to lead one to the unity, to a realization that we are all breathing the same air and that there is only one proprietor who is giving the same vitality to you and me. In the school of meditation, one learns the process that makes one aware of the unity of life within all these multiples. Meditation makes a person aware of oneness, whereas hypnosis makes a person aware of manyness. One unites; the other divides. One is internal; the other is external.

Meditation leads one to the silence within. Most people don't know what silence is. They have never enjoyed it. They may go to a quiet room where there is no outer sound, but the mind remains noisy all the time. Once I told my master that I had observed silence for a long time, that I knew what silence was. He laughed at me and said, "If you don't talk to anybody and put yourself in a pit, do you call it silence? No. That's not true silence. You can take silence anywhere you are if you have developed the power of withdrawal. Then you can be in the midst of the world and yet remain in silence. If you have not done that, then no matter where I put you, you will be disturbed." But silence can cripple one if he is not prepared for it. It can drive a person crazy from unfulfilled cravings for external companionship. How can external silence give one internal silence? The mind will start becoming more active when one is silent externally. But when one learns to love the silence within, then the highest of all joys becomes that deep silence in which one goes beyond all the states of one's mind. The mind then turns within and enjoys that peace beyond.

Preparation for Meditation

Before one is ready for meditation, there are two necessary steps one has to practice. First one should learn to train one's attention, and then one should learn to concentrate: only then can one learn meditation. One should learn to pay attention toward what one does. Many people create great problems for themselves by not paying attention, and this keeps them from enjoying anything. Many people fill up their intestines, they stuff their stomachs full, without paying any attention. But they still feel empty because they have not satisfied their minds. Many people do sex while their minds are somewhere else; they do not know how to enjoy it. Many people do not enjoy a restful sleep because they use this time to be somewhere else in their dreams. Many people, when conversing, habitually say, "Huh? I beg your pardon. What did you say?" because their attention drifts somewhere else. All this dissipation overburdens the mind. Wherever one is physically, whatever one is doing, one should be there mentally also. One should learn to train one's attention.

Then one should develop the ability to concentrate. Concentration is the fruit of the long practice of attention. Concentration is actually very easy: one simply has to sit down and close off the nostrils. Then if one tries to think of many things, it will not be possible—the mind will think only of breathing. This means the mind is very closely related to the breath and that it can be trained with the breath. No matter how much someone loves another person or one's wealth or home, the highest love is the mind wedded with the breath. They are so deeply wedded and committed to each other that they live together all the time. If there is some problem in the mind, it will be reflected in the breath. The highest of all objects for concentration is breath awareness. Once the mind becomes one-pointed, it is a tremendous force. It can create miracles in the world and increase the happiness and well-being of others. A one-pointed mind bestows immense physical, neural, mental, and spiritual benefits.

The States of Consciousness

The school of meditation talks about the body, mind, and spirit in the following way. One has a body, but he is not the body. Then, when one starts observing himself, one comes to know that he is a breathing being also, and then he learns that he is a thinking being too. When one examines his thinking process, one finds that up to a certain period he thinks, and then he starts dreaming and going into a deeper state of unconsciousness called sleep. One experiences three states of mind: waking, dreaming, and sleeping. The conscious waking part of the mind is being trained by our educational system, but there is no systematic education anywhere that trains the unconscious mind, the totality of the mind. So far, most people have been trained and educated to see, watch, and verify things externally, but they do not know how to understand their own internal states.

No one teaches people how to dream or how to sleep or what happens when one dreams and sleeps. So only a small part of mind is being educated by the so-called educational system, and no one teaches whether one can go beyond the three states of waking, dreaming, and sleeping, or how one would feel, what one's condition would be, beyond these three states of mind. If one is not able to go beyond these three states of mind, then one cannot establish a link between the unconscious and the center of consciousness. Meditation is the method that teaches one how to know all these states. So, if one really wants to understand oneself, one should invest some time in meditation. But if one does not understand the method of meditation, one should not pose to sit in meditation and waste one's time and energy. If one merely learns to sit quietly, breathe deeply, and gently allow all one's thoughts to go away, even this will be very helpful and relaxing. Deeper states and higher steps of meditation will lead one to Self-realization, to a higher level of being.

There are two methods for beginning the practice of meditation. One method is to know first and then to tread the path; the other method is to start practicing, and through experience know the truth. The first path says one should gather enough information through books, teachers, seminars, sages, and sayings and then, with doubts dispelled, follow the path that millions have followed before. The other says one should start practicing and let his experience guide him. Both of these paths should be united—one should learn and know, and at the same time practice. No one is fully happy when treading the path of the external world. Yet the path of meditation does not condemn the external path. The external path is full of means, but it is not the end. If one is searching for the end, for fulfillment, by following the external path, then he is searching in the wrong place.

The method of meditation systematically leads one to the source of consciousness through experiencing various levels, one after another. Whenever the mind goes from one experiential state to another, it is a new experience, and the mind will definitely be bewildered and confused. One is already confused, though, so one should not be afraid of the new confusion or want to give up. One should learn to understand all the other levels of consciousness. This path does not promise that one will meet God, because that is a word that has never been analyzed by anybody. People have been wanting this for ages, creating more misery for themselves and having little solace. But they are not trying to understand the Reality. The path of meditation will not give one anything that one does not already have. The path of meditation will lead one to oneself on all levels. People know themselves only on one level, and therefore they think they are small and limited; they are confused and hate themselves. But the path of meditation says this petty self is not the true Self. When one knows the Reality, one knows that there is no difference between the Reality and oneself. One realizes, "I am That."

Breath Awareness and Meditation

From Science of Breath *(1976)*

Breath awareness is an essential part of meditation. The most well established schools of meditation teach breath awareness before leading a student toward an advanced technique of meditation, but some of the modern schools of meditation and relaxation do not understand the importance of breath awareness. In our daily lives we learn to move, but no one teaches us how to be still. This constant habit of movement makes our unconscious habits stronger and stronger, and finally all of our movements are controlled by our unconscious mind. When in the practice of meditation we begin to learn to still our bodies, we become aware of body twitches, tremors, and movements; then, when we begin learning the techniques of breath awareness, we become aware that we can have conscious control over the body, breath, and mind.

All of the exercises of *pranayama,* or breath control, help the student to regulate the motion of the lungs. Without such regulation, the respiratory system, the heart, the brain, and the autonomic nervous system do not function in a balanced way. People commonly assume that the involuntary system cannot be brought under voluntary control, and for the average person this seems true, but those who are accomplished in the art and science of breath control have proved that this assumption is false. The motion of the lungs must be brought under conscious control before advanced techniques of controlling the autonomic nervous system can be attempted.

The science of breath is vital for a student who wants to learn the higher techniques of meditation. When we have learned to sit in a calm, quiet place in a comfortable, steady posture, and body tremors are no longer a source of disturbance, we find four irregularities in the breath: shallowness of breath, jerks in the breath, sounds in the breath, and pauses between inhalation and exhalation. These irregularities disturb the mind and prevent it from concentrating. In the early stages, students practice various methods of breathing in which they use their fingers to close and open the nostrils. We are not going to discuss those breathing exercises here, but one must practice them before practicing breath awareness, which is an advanced technique. Some schools of meditation, such as the Buddhist and Zen schools, do not teach these exercises as do the yoga schools, but for these schools also breath awareness is the most important step for meditation.

In the monastic tradition, teachers do not impart the advanced techniques of meditation unless they see that the student has attained stillness of the body and serenity of the breath. Sitting still is very important—the less movement, the more steady the mind will be. All of the movements, gestures, tremors, and twitchings of the body are caused by an undisciplined and untrained mind. When we examine our behavior, we find that not a single act or gesture is independent of the mind. The mind moves first and then the body moves, and the more the body moves, the more the mind dissipates.

Meditative Discipline

Meditation expands awareness, but this does not mean that awareness should be external. It is a natural tendency of the mind to roam toward the objects of the world. This also can be considered awareness, but such awareness is completely dissipated and gross. The schools of meditation use awareness in a different way. Meditation teaches the student to make the mind one-pointed and inward. To some degree all human beings are aware of their environment and the things related to them. This is the dimmest and most superficial state of human consciousness, and we are not discussing that sort of awareness here. Human consciousness flows through various degrees and grades from the center of consciousness, and systematically going back to the source of consciousness within is the purpose of meditation.

The mind is in the habit of identifying itself with the objects of the world, and it does not become aware of internal states as long as it remains in its dissipated condition. But with meditative discipline, the mind starts traveling inward toward the subtler, finer levels. When one attains a state of perfect stillness and tranquility, that which is beyond the mind reveals itself. Actually, nothing is attained in meditation—a meditator simply allows the Reality to be revealed through a calm and tranquil mind. Tranquility of the mind is an important factor, but more important is breath awareness. The first step in the practice of meditation is a steady, comfortable, and easy posture. The second step is calm, serene, and even breathing. The third is a calm and steady mind; this is the only means for experiencing the deeper levels of being. The fourth step is control of the conscious mind used during the waking state; this control can make one dynamic and creative. In the fifth step, the involuntary system as well as a vast part of the unconscious mind, including the memory, is brought under conscious control. In the sixth step, the mind becomes aware that it is conditioned by time, space, and causation. Through prolonged, unbroken concentration and the regular practice of meditation, the mind can be trained to remain aware of the now, which is an essential part of eternity. This is the seventh step in which a superconscious state full of bliss, peace, happiness, and wisdom is attained.

After serious observation and analysis of the workings of the mind, we find that the mind forms a habit of being conditioned either by remembering past experiences or by imagining future experiences. There is no technique that helps the mind become aware of the now except that of meditation. Meditation is not a method of allowing the mind to roam aimlessly. It is also not something that dawns all of a sudden; it is not an instant method, as some lazy and confused people think. It is a conscious effort of training the body, the breath, and the mind. Meditation should be practiced systematically. No doubt a few visions and unusual experiences are possible by practicing meditation haphazardly, but it is not possible to attain the fruits expected by such methods. If a student practices systematically, it will not take much time for him or her to realize the highest state of bliss.

The Science of Breath

The breath is the bridge or link between the body and the mind. Inhalation and exhalation are the two guards of the city of life. They remain constantly awake doing their duties during all states—waking, dreaming, and sleeping—and their behavior changes instantly according to one's thinking. Inhalation and exhalation are the vehicles through which the *pranas*—vital forces—travel in the living mechanism. There are many other vehicles described by the scriptures that are not important to discuss here, but by close study of the behavior of one's breath, one can discover the subtle functions of these vehicles. The ancient scriptures say that "A pandit [wise person] is one who knows the science of prana." The school of the Pranavedins ("knowers of prana") claims that all the activities of human life can be converted into divinity, but that this is possible only through the mastery of the breath and the prana. There are some books in English available on the subject, though many scriptures remain untranslated. Some of the ancient scriptures say that the pranas are more vital than the mind—"That which moves the mind is also a prana."

The advanced yogis observe that the breath is like a thermometer that registers the conditions of the mind and the influence of the external environment on the body. Many techniques are explained in the book *Shiva Svarodaya.* Those who have studied breath behavior and this science know their mental and physical behavior correctly, and their lives are guided by their control of *svaras,* or life ripples. Our breath behavior can warn us of impending illnesses that might create disturbances in the body. For example, when the body suffers from fever, the nostrils start behaving in a funny way—one of them may start flowing excessively or become blocked. In such a condition, the respiratory system does not function normally; the lungs, heart, and related systems are disturbed, and the mind loses its equilibrium. Advanced yogis also use their breath behavior to watch the capacity of their minds and bodies, and they control the behavior of their breath by various exercises.

Patanjali, the codifier of yoga science, explains in two aphorisms (Yoga Sutras 2:52-53) the spiritual value of pranayama, and he states that we can discipline the mind by practicing the science of breath. Manu, the prominent ancient lawmaker, also recognized prana as one of the important steps in meditation. For hatha yogis, pranayama is also important. According to our school of meditation also, breath awareness is an important step, after establishing a still and comfortable posture, for the awakening of *sushumna*. Although the word *sushumna* cannot be adequately translated into English, it signifies the state of an undisturbed and joyous mind. When the breath starts flowing freely and smoothly through both nostrils, the mind attains this state of joy and calmness. Such a mental condition is necessary for the mind to travel into deeper levels of consciousness, for if the mind is not brought to a state of joy it cannot remain steady, and an unsteady mind is not fit for meditation. Additionally, one of the schools of meditation, which believes in awakening the kundalini, says that without awakening the sushumna, deep meditation and the awakening of kundalini is impossible.

The process of awakening the sushumna is possible only when a student starts enjoying being still by keeping the head, neck, and trunk straight. This means that the student does not allow any uneasiness to occur in the three cords along the spinal column—the central, sympathetic, and parasympathetic ganglionated cords. The moment one starts meditating on the flow of the breath, one starts observing the various defects in its flow—such as noise, shallowness, jerkiness, and that which disturbs one the most, the pause between inhalation and exhalation. Much has been spoken about this in the scriptures, but practice makes one increasingly aware of its importance. When one starts meditating on the flow of the breath, one finds that such a pause distracts the mind. Some of the scriptures say that the pause can be expanded; some say that it can be omitted. In the beginning one has to go through the exercises of pranayama, and particularly the exercises of breath retention. Later one needs more mental effort. Those who do not want to do pranayama exercises can still do meditation, but without breath awareness a deep state of meditation is impossible.

Meditation on the Breath

What should be the object of meditation? Various schools of meditation recommend different objects of focus to make the mind become one-pointed. These objects may be either concrete or abstract—physical objects, sound syllables, mental images, and so on. But none of these objects are helpful in the long run if breath awareness is not practiced. The mind is in the habit of dwelling on images, objects, symbols, ideas, fancies, and fantasies, so merely giving a new object to the mind is not going to enable the practitioner of meditation to transcend the mind.

The breath and the mind are interdependent. If one retains the breath, one's mind starts becoming one-pointed; if the breath is irregular and jerky, the mind is dissipated. After one attains steadiness in one's posture, meditation on the breath or breath awareness is very natural. But when we do not have patience and long to have unusual experiences and to see visions without understanding what we want to visualize and experience, then the mind plays its usual tricks in bringing forward memories and past experiences, mostly in distorted forms. In such cases the mind should not be allowed to hallucinate or experience thought patterns coming from the bed of memory.

An untrained and uncontrolled mind experiences many difficulties in the attempt to become focused and one-pointed. The usual obstacles in the beginning stage of meditation are that the mind habitually runs to old grooves; that it broods on the objects of its interest; and that it feels tired and starts losing consciousness, making the student feel sleepy. But breath awareness strengthens the mind and makes it easier for the mind to become inward. It is advisable for beginners not to worry about any object of meditation but to simply be aware of the breath. This is the simplest, most natural, and most essential step for attaining the deepest state of meditation. Those students who are prepared for an advanced meditational technique realize that breath awareness is important for calming down an agitated mind and making it one-pointed. When the mind starts following the flow of the breath, one becomes aware of the reality that all the creatures of the world are breathing the same breath; that there is a direct communication between oneself and the center of the cosmos, which supplies breath to all living creatures. As long as the center or living unit in human life receives the vital force, or prana, through the breath, the body/mind relationship is sustained. When this communication is disrupted, the conscious mind fails, and the body is separated from the inner unit of life. This separation is called death.

Meditation is a method that helps us to fathom our internal states and finally to go to the source or center of consciousness within. It is a journey within, and if it is practiced systematically it is not difficult at all. Ordinarily the mind remains dissipated with the objects of the world, and so when we try to be still physically we find that our mind roams toward these various worldly objects. Breath awareness helps make our mind one-pointed and inward, thereby enabling us to experience levels that cannot normally be experienced.

India's Contribution to Holistic Health

From Journal of Holistic Health, *April, 1980*

A human being is a citizen of two worlds, the world within and the world outside, but there seems to be a great gap between these two. This gap needs to be bridged, because one-sided progress is not enough—a half-truth is not truth. One who is able to create this bridge between the inner and the external life can be considered to be the perfect person. This is the enterprise of holistic health. Holistic health is a modern, scientific, and systematic approach to living.

There are three categories of people traveling through the procession of life: those who are time-oriented, those who are goal-oriented, and those who are purpose-oriented. Time-oriented people move in the world without understanding why they are moving; they have no true vision of the future. They spend their lives fantasizing about some idyllic future or analyzing triumphs or defeats from the past, failing to appreciate things the way they are. They are thus forever dissatisfied. For such people, staying healthy and finding success is difficult.

Goal-oriented people are those who can physically and mentally discipline themselves to a certain extent. They can conduct their duties according to their circumstances, but their vision remains limited. For lack of higher purpose, their lives remain oriented toward material goals. The third category is composed of those few who are purpose-oriented. Whatever they think, speak, and do is in accordance with their purpose in life.

They regulate their habits and know that physical and mental health are not two different things; they are inseparable units that are essential for maintaining holistic health. For them, maintaining good physical and mental health is like preserving two fine instruments to carry out the purpose of life. What label one attaches to this purpose—happiness, perfection, health, a state of tranquility, nirvana, samadhi, Godhead—is immaterial. The people of this last category are rare, but they are healthy in all respects.

The ancient sages of India emphasized the need for holistic health. They understood the whole being. They understood the interrelationships of body, mind, and consciousness; they knew that the body is merely a covering outside the mind, and that the mind is a covering for the center of consciousness within. It is very important to be aware that the body is merely a tool and not the entire self. However, because the body is a support system for the mind, it is necessary to take proper care of it; if the body is sick, the mind is absorbed by pain and cannot function in a healthy way. Conversely, the mind controls the body. You can easily demonstrate this to yourself. Stop reading for a moment and slowly get out of your chair. Watch carefully. You will soon realize that it is not your body that does the standing; it is something else within that orders the mass of flesh and bones to stand. The body is merely an instrument that obeys orders. The center that gives the orders has the potential to be one's greatest ally or one's worst enemy—the source of health or of disease.

How does one maintain good physical and mental health so that the purpose of life can be carried out? There are practices that have been taught in the yoga tradition for many centuries. These are not just physical, they are mental and spiritual, too, for yoga is the science of self-effort, of self-examination, and of self-awareness. It is a scientific discipline perfected over millennia. The yoga techniques work; they have been proven and validated. By sincerely and honestly following these simple guidelines and exercises, one will achieve success. As one practices, he or she will begin to see and feel how much has been accomplished through self-effort, and in this way will understand the way to further attainment.

Cleansing and Nourishing

The ancient yoga manuscripts describe two sets of mechanisms in the human body: one for cleansing the body, the other for nourishing it. They work together in harmony, balancing each other. The yoga manuals first make one aware of the four major excretory systems that cleanse the body: the lungs, pores, kidneys, and bowels. So one should watch and see that the lungs expand rhythmically, that the pores are functioning properly, that the kidneys are operating normally, and that the bowels move regularly. One should try to understand one's natural cleansing systems and learn to control and assist them, because if these systems are not functioning properly, the nourishing systems cannot do their work properly, and the body begins to break down. Resistance and irregularity create disorders and disease. The mind then remains under stress, and the nervous system remains in tension.

According to the ancient texts, there are a few very simple exercises designed to maintain the strength of the body's excretory systems. Although all practices mentioned in the manuals are important, the most important are those that have to do with regulating the motion of the lungs. That is why you should practice breathing exercises. Breathing is more important than eating, for the breath is the bridge between mind and body; it is also the subtle thermometer that registers the conditions of both body and mind. The breath is also a vehicle for the energy called *prana*. Inhalation and exhalation constantly function like two caretakers in the City of Life. The exhalation expels the used-up gases, and the inhalation supplies the vital energy—oxygen and prana—from the atmosphere.

The lungs work in the body like the flywheel of a machine, and if you learn to regulate the breath, you will be able to control their motion. So you should start by practicing diaphragmatic breathing. The diaphragm is a dome-shaped muscle located under the lungs. One inhales by contracting, or pulling down, the diaphragm, and this forces the abdomen outward and sucks air into the lungs. Relaxing the diaphragm allows it to float up to its original position, and when this happens the air is expelled. Breathing diaphragmatically may be one of the most important of all conscious acts. It is certain to produce a sense of tranquility and to reduce stress and tension, thus adding years to a person's life.

There are four basic things to watch for in learning to breathe properly. First, learn to fill the lungs fully with each breath, for in breathing deeply, we use our full lung capacity. Slowly, you will find this capacity increasing. Second, as you practice breathing you should be sure not to create long pauses between the inhalation and the exhalation. This is very important. At the Himalayan Institute, research has revealed that anyone who creates a long pause after expiration is predisposed to the development of coronary disease. The third thing to observe is the regular flow of inhalation and exhalation. The breath should be smooth, for when it flows smoothly, relaxation can take place; when it is irregular the body cannot rest. The last thing to watch for is noisy breathing. This is a sign of obstruction in the nostrils, and if it is allowed to continue, you may start inhaling through the mouth, which is not healthy as a normal practice.

After you learn to breathe properly, you will find that your thinking has become very clear. In addition, when you have learned to regulate your lungs by eliminating shallowness, pauses, jerks, and noise, you have done your work as far as cleansing the lungs is concerned.

Along with cleansing techniques, the ancients also stressed the importance of knowing about a balanced and nutritious diet. There is no one diet that is perfect for all. Every person is unique, for each has a different metabolism. However, there are some general guidelines that apply to almost everyone. For instance, one should choose unprocessed, unrefined, whole foods without artificial chemicals, and one should not eat excessive amounts of sugar and salt.

As described in the ancient manuals, food falls into two

different categories: cleansers and nourishers. Fruits have a high cleansing value, while vegetables, grains, legumes, and dairy products have a high nourishing value. Both types of food should be included in the diet. There should also be a balance of solids and liquids. For most people, the diet should consist of about forty percent whole grains, twenty percent beans, twenty percent vegetables, fifteen percent fruits and raw vegetables, and five percent dairy products. Although there are advantages to following a vegetarian diet, it is not necessary to do this in order to lead a spiritual life. But it is important to eat in a spirit of calm. The ancients cooked their food and ate it as an offering to God who created it for them, and for those who understand that secret of life, their day-to-day life becomes an act of worship.

Being Still

It is only after you have learned to take care of your body that you can tread the path of inner life. Proper nourishing and cleansing are the prerequisites for the next step in the cultivation of health: being still. The ancients found that by sitting in a steady, comfortable position, one frees oneself from the distractions of the body and is able to attend to the mind. For this reason, you must discipline yourself to a regular and consistent habit of sitting in order to counteract the pressure of bad habits which keep the body under stress. In the beginning, the body may send messages saying that it is unwilling to do this, and so you must cultivate patience; it is best to increase your capacity slowly and gradually. You should observe but not condemn yourself.

When the physical body begins to become still, the mind becomes more active. If you maintain your stillness, you will become able to observe your thoughts as they emerge, and you will slowly contact and calm the conscious mind and body. At this point it is very helpful to practice breath awareness, because the breath is closely related to the conscious mind. They are, in fact, interdependent; you can train and regulate the mind by being aware of your breathing. So let the mind be aware of the breath and watch how it flows. If you can do this for three minutes—only three minutes without any diversion—it will bring good results.

Then you must understand yourself from within. Doing so allows you to develop the ability to choose the best alternatives, to practice discrimination. Then, once you have learned how to analyze a situation and to decide what to do, it is necessary to be determined to carry it out, to exercise will power. The final step in this progress is proper action. There is a Sanskrit word, *apta,* which means "one who does and says whatever he or she thinks." This is important, because self-reliance comes from the performance of actions. So through regular practice, patience, observation, analysis, discrimination, determination, and proper action, the mind becomes concentrated, and a concentrated mind can meditate very nicely. Through perseverance in meditation, one at last reaches the state of samadhi, the state of tranquility in which one does things, yet remains above them. Then as one's consciousness goes to the height of samadhi, one's wisdom increases until complete transformation to a state of perfection takes place. This is the state of perfect stillness.

Allowing Reality to Flow

Once we turn within and start understanding our internal states, making the mind one-pointed, we become aware of the fact that the emotional level is deeper than the level of thoughts. It is therefore necessary to develop emotional power. The emotions have their source in *kama,* the prime desire, the mother of all emotions, the primary cause of all motivations. Actions are performed according to the types of one's desire, but all actions arise from four primitive fountains: self-preservation, sleep, food and sex. If these four primitive fountains are controlled, they can be the source of good health and longevity. Control of these fountains leads to the ability to regulate the thinking processes, and to mastery over all the emotions. If, however, these fountains are not regulated, they will be the source of many problems and diseases.

When we study the emotions, we find that there are seven main streams of negative emotions that arise from the four primitive fountains or appetites. Desire, or *kama,* is the first stream and the mother of all the others. Anger, pride, attachment, greed, jealousy, and egoism are the other six streams. By studying our thoughts, speech, and actions, however, we can attain emotional maturity. The emotions can then be controlled by regulation and balance according to our capacity. Then, when the four primitive urges are regulated and the seven streams of emotion are controlled, the positive emotions emerge. These lead to self-reliance and self-confidence; they motivate mind, action, and speech in a joyous and creative way. Unselfish love is the highest positive emotion; it can lead to devotion, for when one loves another, one wants to serve and give to the beloved. Unselfish love also leads to joy, peace, tranquility, and equilibrium. Emotion is truly a great power, provided it is directed and applied in a positive way.

All human beings want to attain a state of happiness that is free from pains and fears, and this can be attained by practicing self-training. The ancients described such a program in the traditional yoga manuscripts, a program that provides us with a way to reach a state of health on all levels. In following it, we learn through direct experience, for that alone is valid; it can be challenged by no one. Self-training for self-knowledge works through direct experience, and although it is very subtle, it can bring a person to the finest possible level of understanding. It is the best of all therapies. We must first begin by practicing spirituality in our day-to-day life, using our own free will and being honest with ourselves. After this, we should learn detachment. This means that we should be of the world but remain above, no matter what happens. To maintain tranquility, we must be constantly aware of our goal.

There are two techniques that can help us do this. The first is to become self-reliant. Happiness can never be given by anyone; happiness comes through the right attitude of mind. It comes out of an internal state of tranquility that allows us to go through the procession from the known to the unknown without disturbance. The second technique that can help us remain aware of the Reality within while doing actions in the world is internal dialogue. One should sit down every morning and talk with oneself. This prepares us for meditational therapy, which, if used and understood properly, is the highest of all therapies. It teaches us how to be still and how to be free from the stress created by suppressions and repressions. Through it, we can strengthen our positive thinking patterns and become emotionally mature. Then by allowing the unconscious mind to come forward, we can go beyond it: the inner Reality can come to the conscious field and expand. We cannot explore the totality of the mind unless we apply the special technique called meditation; unless we use that inward method, we will never be able to understand ourselves within. We will not be able to communicate, to relate to the external world, or to use our intelligence in a creative way. This ability comes through involving ourselves in a self-training program.

How do we realize that Reality which is beyond names and forms? When our mind is prepared for it, then we will start treading the path of spirituality and start enlightening ourselves. Enlightenment comes through direct experience from within. It is not a creation; it is not an attainment. How do we know what enlightenment is? We know because great people who were born just like us, whose mothers were just like our mothers, who walked on the earth, who were human beings, but who also had enlightenment, have told us what it is and how to reach it. Human beings do not understand that they are complete, so they should learn to believe, appreciate, and admire their own existence first. That is what proves the reality of the existence of the Lord. My master used to say, "You are already God, so don't try to know God. That godly part is already there in you. All you have to do is become fully human. That is your part to play—to be a good human being so that the reality called God can flow spontaneously."

Enlightenment is an expansion of consciousness. When we become enlightened, we become aware of something more than ourselves, of something more than our own interests. The more we become aware of others, the closer we come to the center where we find a unity underlying all diversity. There are many waves, but there is only one water. All human beings are different, but they all inhale and exhale the same life force. If we want truth to be revealed to us, it will be, but first we have to create the proper conditions. If you were to go to a powerhouse with a light bulb in your hand and ask, "Will you please light my bulb?" it could not do it. The power outlet is within you. You are shouting, "O powerhouse, O powerhouse, please come to me!" But it's already there.

Religion and Science in the Future of Humanity

Presented to the International Conference of Scientists and Religious Leaders on Shaping the Future of Mankind, Kyoto, Japan, July 17-21, 1978

What am I? What is this universe? Are there realities beyond the reach of our senses? What is my relationship with the universe? These are some of the questions both religion and science have investigated ever since human beings discovered that their intelligence is aware of itself. When human intelligence first discovered the pronoun *I*, it declared the human capacity to recognize oneself as a special entity; each individual proclaiming *I* feels himself or herself to be special in the universe. Thus we enter into an inquiry about our relationship with the universe.

Originally, inquiring minds were not divided into the followers of either religion or science. Those great beings who tried to answer the basic questions of life did not completely separate the various areas of knowledge. Rather, they had the realization that the fundamental answers to these questions could be found only by first finding out the nature of intelligence. Thus they probed into the depths of their own consciousness and discovered that all consciousness is One and that it permeates the universe. The great philosophers, prophets, and saints have declared this truth throughout the millennia of human civilization among all cultures, countries, and religions.

The most important part of their teachings regarding the nature of the universe is that the world of matter cannot be understood without first discovering the depths of this inner consciousness. These masters never denied the importance of

171

understanding the external reality of the universe, but they insisted that we must first understand the nature of *I* by looking into ourselves in deep contemplation, by diving into our depths. There, all philosophers of ancient religions agree. In the Vedas they declared, "I am the first-born son of Eternal Truth." We read in the Upanishads: "As though lightning flashed, such is the moment when great Brahman becomes known." In the Bhagavad Gita, Krishna showed to Arjuna the *Virat,* the cosmic expanse of the great consciousness, on the battlefield of Kurukshetra. Lao-Tsu, the Buddha, and all the other founders of great systems of philosophy moved their disciples' minds by conveying similar truth. Likewise, the prophets of the Old Testament have repeatedly testified to hearing and seeing God's voice and vision.

When the prophets spoke in such powerful voices, their words seemed to come from a source very different from that of their listeners. A river of inspiration carried their listeners' minds. Those who heard could not help themselves but intuitively believed that, indeed, the great *siddhas, buddhas,* and *muktas*— the adepts, the enlightened ones, the free ones—were speaking from oceanic depths far beyond the shallow surfaces of intelligence that ordinary human beings explore.

Those who doubt often ask believers, How can we rationally accept that such words of the masters are true? But I say, How can we not accept it, when many witnesses in all parts of the world at different times have testified to the same reality in similar words? Were they insane? Was the Buddha insane to sit absolutely still for forty-nine days to reach enlightenment? What insane person can sit still for even forty-nine seconds? The words of Jesus have been reverberating around this planet for the past two thousand years. Why not also the words of all the billions of others who call themselves sane? Indeed, the power behind the words of the founders of religions comes from a reservoir that can be found in all of us as we probe deep into our own intelligence and consciousness to unravel the meaning of *I.*

Those disciples who heard the words of their masters seldom understood them. They tried to comprehend the masters' words by guesswork, without themselves going deeply enough into the experience of inner exploration through contemplation and meditation. Through this guesswork, many disciples tried to interpret the words of the masters in various ways. This caused disagreements, and thus many different systems of belief arose and became religions. In this way the paths of religion eventually became separated from true spirituality. When the experience of inner reality is personal, it is spiritual. But when someone states that he believes that someone else has had an unnamed experience, then he is following a religion.

Science and Spirituality

When we are primarily concerned with the nature of the universe apart from our intelligence, it becomes science; when intelligence tries to understand its own nature, it becomes spirituality. Religion and science may disagree, but science and spirituality cannot disagree because both are experiential. Science explains the nature of the non-*I*—what it is that we do not identify with our intelligence. Spirituality unravels the mystery of the *I*. Between the *I* and the non-*I* there is a link. This link is called the mind. The mind borrows from the inner *I* a semblance of intelligence and extends it outward. It also gathers the experiences of the external world and conveys them to the deeper inner intelligence. It is for this reason that the yogis understand the realities of the universe by looking directly into their own minds, as there is no part or particle of the universe that is not pervaded by the cosmic mind. The contribution of spirituality and religion to science needs to be remembered in this context. The great spiritual leaders were the first scientists.

The yogis have found that the scientific principles that govern the universe are not entirely separate from the principles that govern the mind. It is thus that the spiritual traditions of the ancient past gave birth to a great many sciences. The greatest philosophers of Greece inquired both into the nature of intelligence and into the non-intelligent universe, and they became the founders of scientific inquiry in Western civilization.

The yogis developed highly advanced principles of arithmetic and geometry simply by experiencing the patterns that brain waves create. When these patterns are projected out from the experiencing mind, they become points, lines, and triangles. Who can say whether the highly accurate designs employed in composing mandalas are scientific or spiritual? Is the construction of altars to represent mandalas an exercise in science or a mental experience of the devotee and worshiper? Are temples, pyramids, and churches—which are three-dimensional representations of mandalas, which, again, are projections of brain-wave patterns— part of an expression of an inner experience, or an experiment with architectural design?

The yogis sent their minds probing into the intricate energy and *prana* patterns of their own personalities and not only came up with the energy maps of the body but also discovered the basis of anatomy. When they tuned themselves to the sounds of the musical rhythms produced by brain-wave patterns, they found that these fine patterns themselves were grosser modulations of yet finer modes of a music that is played by and within the cosmic mind. They found that the notes of these sounds and energy waves were part of a point/counterpoint juxtaposition of the rhythms of duality that developed from the one thought that is the universe. Thus the sound and energy waves become atoms—points of energy that are called *shakti-bindu*. When the mind is highly concentrated on a single point, a *bindu*, then all the points and counterpoints of the universe are immediately understood.

Without the aid of modern telescopes, the yogis of India asserted that there are as many worlds as there might be hairs on the body of God. The ancient yogis may not have developed a highly complex technology in modern terms, because their contribution to humanity was in a different direction; but it is now well known that yogis are capable of demonstrating in experimental situations facts that baffle the scientists of today. For centuries, the works of science such as mathematics, astronomy, and medicine were preserved in the monasteries of all religions, and the monks were the first astronomers and surgeons. The Arab founders of Western medicine like Ibn-Sina (Avicenna) found no conflict between discussing the nature of angels on the one hand and establishing medical colleges on the other. To unite that which appears diverse to others' eyes, the yogis have stated from the time of the Upanishads, "There are no diversities in the universe; all is a single infinite expanse known as Brahman."

A Whole with Two Parts

Those on the path of yoga are often mistaken as being in the same class as followers of various religions, churches, sects, and cults whose believers (though not the ancient founders) are incapable of scientifically demonstrating the truth of their beliefs. Now, today much endeavor is put into holding a dialogue between science and religion. In the ancient texts, it is said that there can be two kinds of dialogue between experts. One is called *sandhaya-sambhasha*—a dialogue between friendly seekers who are trying to arrive at a single truth by matching and joining two opposite pieces of a complete picture. The second is called *vigrihya-sambhasha*—a discussion between rivals, each asserting that his own piece is the complete picture, or that the half of the picture held by the other is somehow inferior and subservient.

We read in the Bhagavad Gita that human intelligence operates on three levels. On the lowest level, it sees a part of something and considers that to be the complete whole. On the second level, it gathers many parts and tries to create a complete whole by joining them together. At the highest level, it sees the complete whole first, and thereby comprehends all its parts. This last is the purest level of intelligence. So the yoga tradition views spirituality and science to be two parts of a complete whole. The future of mankind will be secure when the antagonistic views held by dogmatic scientists and dogmatic religious leaders are finally wedded together—not as though two opponents were declaring a truce, but as though two hands were obeying the commands of a single brain.

Both science and spirituality are primarily experiences within the principle of intelligence. As I have said already, when intelligence inquires into its own nature, it becomes spirituality. Here we are not talking of intellectual inquiry or philosophical speculation, because this is entirely guesswork. Thousands of philosophers have created hundreds of encyclopedic works based on such speculation without any inner experience. They cannot agree among themselves, and they create confusion and conflict among their readers and followers. Their language primarily relates to external realities and cannot convey the experience of the oceanic vastness of that dimension of intelligence that the founders of spirituality have experienced. The founders of true spirituality agree on the nature of their inner experience, but the mere speculative philosophers continue to disagree (unless, in rare cases like Socrates and Kant, speculation gives way to allow transcendental silence to flow through). The same applies to the speculative theologian, who ventures elaborate and complicated guesswork as to the true meaning of the words spoken by the founders of the traditions. Quite often such guesswork has been falsely given the name of contemplation, not realizing that true contemplation is, once again, a silent experience. Neither the philosopher nor the theologian has any business pretending to proclaim a truth without first coming face to face with the deeper nature of intelligence, where consciousness goes far beyond the triangle of space, time, and causation.

I wish to reassert that science, too, is an experience of a spiritual intelligence, but in relationship to the external universe. In the Upanishads we are told that the Transcendent, *Shukla Brahman*, is pure intelligence, *Prajnanam*, but that God seen as immanent in the universe, *Shabala*, is also a reality, the principle of intelligence projected into the universe. To paraphrase Einstein, science studies the manner in which the transcendental intelligence manages the immanent intelligence—how God beyond runs the sacred universe here and now. Thus we find that some of the basic laws taught by both scientists and spiritual teachers are common to all the sciences. Without understanding these cosmic laws, we would fail to perceive the true relationship between the two facets of reality. For example, take Newton's third law of motion: for every motion in one direction, there is an equal motion in the opposite direction. On the spiritual path, this becomes the law of karma: for every action in one direction, there is a reaction in the opposite direction. The wording is different, but the principle is the same. By applying our understanding of Newton's principle, we steer our boats or pilot our jet planes. Through an understanding of the karmic principle, we know that what we do to others is actually a seed being sown in our own minds in the form of subtle impressions, which will ripen later for us to reap. We need to emphasize that the principles of science are applications of spiritual truths, for the universe is an emanation of the Divine Intelligence. Indeed, every scientific thought occurs within the human mind, which is activated by a spark of the Divine Intelligence.

Unity Within Diversity

To understand fully the relationship between science and spirituality, we need to know how the unity and the multiplicity of the universe are intertwined. Every physicist knows that worldly objects exist and operate on many levels of reality at once, as though these many facets were occupying the same space and time and presenting to our poor, limited senses a display of mutually exclusive and contradictory aspects of existence all at once. The ancient Jaina philosophers thought of light as atomic; others viewed it as energy. Today we know that light is both a vibration and a photon, depending on how we view it. Thus, the earlier efforts of science to define everything as a one-level reality have met with abysmal failure. Those who have unraveled the secrets of the world of spirituality have also stated that each level of reality has its own internally valid and self-consistent laws of existence and operation. The rules that apply to drawing an equilateral triangle on a flat surface do not apply on a curved surface, yet one set of rules is not false while the other is true. There are nights and there are days, as well as dawns and dusks in between, and they are all facets of the same reality of time and planetary motions. Parallel lines are defined as two lines at equal distance that cannot meet, and yet we are told that they do meet in infinity. Similarly, science and spirituality meet in infinity. If science had no basis in spirituality, the intuitive flashes of scientific principles that often occur to true seekers of knowledge would not take place. All knowledge arises from deep within the principle of intelligence, or consciousness.

Sages such as Lao-Tsu, Socrates, and the *rishis* of the Upanishads have all said that the infinite is the source of the finite, and that the One and the many are not opponents—the many dwell within the One as the latter's potentialities. They emanate from that One, and after displaying the magic show of the world of *maya*, they all return to Mother Infinity in the One. Spirituality experiences the oneness, while science observes the procedures in the many and their interrelationships within units. It is as though a single unitary point of consciousness expands out and contracts within. The whole universe dwells within a point of intelligence, from which it evolves and to which it returns. Science studies the procedures of the evolution of the multiple universe, while spirituality experiences the innermost One. Unfortunate is the scientist who stakes his entire being on one small unit from amongst the multiples. Fortunate is the seeker of spirituality who will not see the multiples except within the One. We read in the Upanishads: "From death to death goes he who sees as though there were many here," "The Vast is the happiness, there is no happiness in the limited," "Worship the Infinite Vast." Science centering itself only upon isolated units of the multiple will lead humankind from destruction to destruction. Medical science that studies an organ in complete isolation from the entire human personality is not science at all. These sciences have to return to their historical spiritual origins for a greater vision of humanity and the universe.

Today we hear scientists talk about the principles of synergy, and we hear psychologists speak of synchronicity. What these words express is a seeking for the One within the many. All energies that flow in the universe—in a single human cell, within an atomic particle, in the gigantic hearts of the distant suns, and in the vast masses of gases from which the galaxies are yet to be formed—are all interrelated. If the energy of a single atomic particle were lost, the whole structure of the principles on which the universe is built would crumble and vanish.

Though human sciences declare these principles on an intellectual level, we fail to walk with a cosmic consciousness because physical sciences can only state the facts as observed—they cannot create a state of consciousness, they cannot convey the feeling of this unity to human intelligence. If a mind is trained only to deal with the multiples, it will take much forgetting and purifying to develop an intuitive grasp of unity that is infinity. It is true that the spiritual inquiries of the ancients led to the discoveries of sciences; it has also been said that scientific inquiry can lead to spiritual seeking. We hear today's astronomers and physicists proclaim repeatedly that what they study seems to them to be a mystery play of the physical universe that must have a metaphysical author. They guess it to be so but do not know for certain. The same intuitive processes that have helped them often to discover scientific principles can also bring a spiritual realization when developed further. A very ancient dialogue occurs in the Vedas: "Believe in God, if indeed he is, but where is he? Who has seen him?" "Open your eyes and see. Right here before you I am shining in my full glory in every object you behold." The scientist explores the object; the spiritual seeker looks at the glory.

The future of humanity must be seen from both ends. On one end are the means for physical comfort, nourishment, and health of the body, transportation, communications, and our insatiable curiosity about every atomic particle in every galaxy. On the other end is the very nature of humankind, independent of the physical universe. On one extreme, what can a person accomplish without any tools? On the other extreme, what can one accomplish without inner mastery? Though one may be able to explore outer space, can one dive into the spaces within? Can the scientist control his irritations, angers, frustrations? Can he lengthen the duration of his breath to accomplish the dream of a long life? Can he, without any medicines or injections but merely by using the control of his own volition, stop his heartbeat or place himself in suspended animation? Can he teach the individual politician to be at peace within his mind? Can he bring about a peaceful state of mind among the citizens of the world without the use of pills or physiological manipulation? To all these the answer is no. Nor can the spiritual seeker bring nourishment to hungry stomachs without the help of agricultural scientists. To repeat a cliche: without science, humanity is a cripple; without spirituality, it is blind.

We must trace the origin of the intellectual processes on which science depends to their home, the unitary point of intuition. We must acknowledge that intuition, too, diversifies itself into intellectual processes, which return again to their spiritual homeland in states of deep contemplation and meditation. If it depends on science alone, humanity will become so attached to physical objects that insatiable curiosity combined with unsatisfied greed will lead to our destruction in a very short time. Even now, thousands of living species are becoming extinct, and beautiful rain forests are being converted into deserts. The spiritual ways of life of many ancient cultures have been disturbed and irretrievably lost. Through spirituality, the higher intelligence will prevail. Need, but not greed, will be fulfilled, and the present restlessness of masses upon masses of minds poisoning the collective unconscious of this planet will cease its agitations. Guided by pure consciousness, science will serve humanity, while spirituality itself will help raise human relationships to a highly unselfish level of fulfillment.

This is no empty promise. It can be so. This prophecy will be fulfilled. Let science return to its holistic origins, let the scientist remember that it was not for nothing that the monk was the first astronomer and surgeon. Let the scientist today also learn in depth what a swami has to say, and the future of humanity is bright. To the people of religions we have to say: abandon the verbosity of your theologies and preachings from the pulpit; return yourself and your followers to the origins of spirituality, the inner conscious experience of dwelling in the infinite light that is God. Cease this incessant talk about God and seek to meet and know God personally.

Meditation in Christianity

From Meditation in Christiantiy, *1973*

Religion should not consist of mere intellectual conformity. The human mind is badly crippled by thinking that truth has already been found and that nothing remains for us except to reproduce the same beliefs over and over. Religion is the fulfillment of life; it is an experience in which every aspect of being is raised to its highest state. What is needed to attain this, however, is not dogma; it is a change of consciousness, a rebirth, an inner revolution. There is no such thing as the automatic evolution of humanity; evolution is possible only through conscious effort. As they are human beings, they remain unfinished beings. They must seek their own completion. People have to grow into regenerate beings and allow the Christ consciousness to flow through them. This is the teaching of Christianity.

Jesus asks us to bring about this rebirth, but it can take place only through higher knowledge and meditation, not through external living habits or vocal prayer alone. When Jesus rebukes the Pharisees, for instance, he is condemning the man of pretenses who keeps up appearances. "Except your righteousness shall exceed the righteousness of the scribes and Pharisees," he said, "ye shall in no wise enter the kingdom of Heaven" (Matt. 5:20). In other words, to attain heaven (which is the higher level of understanding) one has to grow, and this comes about through prayer, purity, self-control, studying life, and meditation. Christ and Buddha, for instance, freed themselves from the restricting

spread the universal gospel of truth, love, and service.

Jesus says of John the Baptist that he is the best of those born of women but that the least of the kingdom of heaven was greater than he. For example, John speaks to us of salvation through moral life; he tells us what to do, but he does not tell us how to be. Jesus insists on inner transformation. John asks us to become better; Jesus asks us to become new. John the Baptist was puzzled when he heard that Jesus and His disciples drank wine and did not fast. He could not understand it when they plucked the ears of corn on the Sabbath day or when Jesus healed on the Sabbath. John is still a man born of woman; he has not experienced rebirth. Jesus tells us, "Except a man be born again he cannot see the kingdom of God" (John 3:3), and Paul says, "Awake, thou that sleepest and arise from the dead" (Eph. 5:14). Originally, Christian teachings— before they became externalized and dogmatized—focused on awakening from sleep through the light shed by inner wisdom. Jesus Christ was one who had done this and who taught others the way.

Religion is not theology, and it is not magic or witchcraft. It should not spoil the simplicity of truth. Religion is not limited to the data of perception or introspection; it is an experience to be lived, not a theory or belief to be accepted. When a person surrounds his soul with a shell, such as national pride or the empty presumptions of dogma, he suppresses the breath of the spirit. Christianity, on the other hand, is a liberating power that is based on the life and experience of Jesus. The cross becomes significant when we make it our own and undergo crucifixion. Only then can we experience rebirth. "Seek and you shall find" (Matt. 7:7), said Jesus, but each of us must seek independently. The truth that is latent in every soul must become manifest. Then shall we be able to work in newness of life. "Marvel not that I have said unto thee, 'Ye must be born again'" (John 3:7). In this spirit, says St. Paul, ". . . Know ye not that ye are the temple of God and that the spirit of God dwelleth in you? . . . You are the temple of the living God" (I Cor. 3:16-17). One who enters inwardly penetrates intimately into himself and, going beyond self, becomes perfect.

In early Christianity meditation was practiced in all the monasteries, and the cross, a symbol for physical suffering, mortification, and earthly defeat, was also a symbol for spiritual victory. Through suffering lies the way of liberation. Pascal says that Jesus struggles with death until the end of the world, and in this boundless Gethsemane that is the universe, we have to struggle on unto death, wherever a tear falls, wherever a heart is seized with despair, wherever an injustice or an act of violence is committed. "Hast thou seen thy brother, then thou hast seen God." This, the motto of the early Christians, is just as valid to us today.

The Christian Tradition of Meditation

Scriptural witness to meditation pervades both the Old Testament and the Gospels. For instance, in the Psalms one reads:

> Let the words of my mouth and the meditation of my heart be acceptable in they sight, O Lord, my rock and my redeemer. (Psalm 19:14)

> Be still, and know that I am God. (Psalm 46:10)

> Let me hear what God the Lord will speak . . . to those who turn to him in their hearts. (Psalm 85:8)

> I commune with my heart in the night; I meditate and search my spirit. (Psalm 77:6)

> May my meditation be pleasing to him, for I rejoice in the Lord. (Psalm 104:34)

> On the glorious splendor of thy majesty, and on thy wondrous works, I will meditate. (Psalm 145:5)

Further witness of meditation in Christianity can be found in the New Testament, which frequently shows Jesus retiring from the crowds to be alone in meditation, urging his followers to seek the "Father" within. Furthermore, St. Paul's Epistles describe the process of unfolding and inner transformation as one progresses on the path of Christ consciousness. These are but a few instances, among hundreds in the Bible, that clearly reflect the inner experiences of the higher nature. Somewhere, however, the thread between early and modern Christianity was broken—especially regarding the tradition of meditation—and that is the reason why the modern Christian does not receive initiation in meditation. It is also one of the reasons why many people are dissatisfied with the Christian religion as it is known today. Its practical aspect— meditation—is missing.

Meditation is the means for developing the inner life, and this has been reaffirmed by the acknowledged mystics of Christianity. For example:

> Our meditation in this present life should be in the praise of God; for the external exultation of our life hereafter will be the praise of God: and none can become fit for the future life who hath not practiced himself for it now. (St. Augustine)

> Let me know myself, Lord, and I shall know Thee. (St. Augustine)

> No one can be saved without self-knowledge. (St. Bernard)

> Let us enter the cell of self-knowledge. (St. Catherine of Siena)

The above quotations, if deeply studied and properly understood, reveal that in the long line of Christian sages the practice of meditation was more essential than verbal prayer.

Many admirers of Christian mysticism may acknowledge the testimony of mystics but characterize these individuals as exceptional, their experiences beyond the potential of modern seekers. This pessimism endures because Western Christians are not aware of an overlooked tradition, one in which meditation was taught widely. The meditative tradition at one time dominated early Christianity in the Middle East. After studying the history of the early Christians and the Desert Fathers, we know that they meditated day and night, and that meditation was not a new concept for them. Regardless of whether Abba, Paul, or St. Anthony was the first monk and father of the desert, it is quite certain that St. Anthony established a school of very systematic meditation in A.D. 310. It was situated on a mountain, called St. Anthony, sixty-five miles south of Cairo, and there he guided thousands of monks on the path of meditation. Another monastery, the monastery of Tabenna in upper Egypt, was founded by Paul in A.D. 300. According to historical data, Paul was born a few years before the close of the third century, and later in his life he guided monks in practices similar to those of the school of St. Anthony. His school also endorsed the practice of silence.

In all, there were about five thousand monks practicing meditation and austerity in the Desert of Nitra, or the Nitron Valley, in Egypt around that time, and during the second half of the fourth century a large number of ascetics lived all around Cairo. Christianity began to replace the myths and gods of Egypt, and the sign of the cross was often seen instead of the ancient symbols.

To further trace the history of meditation in the West, it is mentioned in various scriptures that two monks from India accompanied Alexander the Great to the Middle East and established a school of meditation in the general region where Anthony and Paul had founded their monasteries. History shows that early Eastern Christianity had a long line of sages, competent in the art of meditation, and comparative studies reveal that their ascetic practices were very similar to, or the same as, those practiced by Indian monks and sages. There is no doubt in my mind that the fathers of the desert and of Mt. Athos, as well as St. Anthony, knew the methods of meditation. This was also the time when Patanjali's school of meditation was influencing the various sects and religions of the Far- and Middle East. Unfortunately, Western Christianity has never seriously absorbed this genuine meditative tradition.

It is also interesting to note that yogic breathing was practiced in the fifth century A.D. by the Hesychast monks. In addition, the spiritual writings of the Hesychastic period teach that the human body has certain focal points that correspond to the *chakras* of yoga—the navel, the heart, the throat, and the mid-brow. The Hesychast monks, like the yogis, would concentrate upon these points in conjunction with rhythmic breathing and prayerful words, and by learning to control the respiration, the aspirant reached a tranquil state and tasted previously unknown spiritual experiences. According to the Hesychasts and the yogis, a transformation of character was gradually produced as one progressed in the art of meditative breathing and the accompanying necessary ascetic practices. Disruptive feelings, ill thoughts, and uncontrollable actions were gradually tranquilized by the steady practice of holy breathing (yogic breathing).

Later, during the Middle Ages, the confluence of Hesychastic prayer and meditation continued to prevail in Christian monasteries, and the great Byzantine mystic St. Simeon (949-1022), practiced and taught these methods of meditation (see *Orientalia Christiana*). One also finds the theory of breathing and the mystic physiology (called *sushumna dhyanam* in yogic manuals) in some modern spiritual treatises that relate breathing to various meditative states.

In addition, two orders who claim to have their own unbroken traditions—the Rosicrucians and the Freemasons—provide us with evidence to suggest a similar connection with yoga. These two orders are very close and often work together, and one finds in their esoteric and mystical histories living testimonials to the fact that they used the symbol for what the yogis consider to be the mother sound, *OM*. For reference one can go through lectures on Masonic symbolism written by the late Grand Master Albert Pike, who explains that *OM* was converted into Egyptian symbols:

> Coleman (*Mythology of the Hindus*) says that Om is a mystic symbol signifying the supreme God of Gods, which the Hindus, from its lawful and sacred meaning, hesitate to pronounce aloud, and in doing so place one of their hands before their mouths. . . .

Understanding the Path of Meditation

The systematic practice of meditation within a definite and accepted metaphysical framework is congenial to all religious schools of the world, for their goal is the same—to bring the aspirants to the highest state of consciousness. Without sufficient understanding of how and why meditation should be practiced, the meditative process cannot lead to this highest state, but if the process is properly understood on all levels, there will be inner peace and a unique experience of profound harmony along the way. In attempting to achieve this meditative experience, however, the aspirant is sooner or later threatened by two restrictions. The first is that the aspirant naturally tends to remain within the traditional boundaries of his accepted metaphysical and religious beliefs. This is the biggest obstacle. The second restriction is that the orthodox methods of meditation prescribed by Hindus, Buddhists, Jews, or Christians discourage people from moving outside their own meditative approach.

Every theological system requires its followers to believe in a definite way, with definite notions of God, soul, heaven, hell, sin, and virtue. But any pre-determined notions that one carries to the deeper states of meditation binds the meditator and prevents him from crossing the boundaries of the conditioned mind. One can receive higher experiences from this kind of meditation, but they are limited. Consequently, when one is restricted by dogma, one cannot realize the universal truth that the Self within is the Self of all. This enlightenment remains far away from the vision of such a meditator.

To tread the path of enlightenment, it is therefore important for the meditator to fully understand a few terms that are often confusing. The first concept is that of evil. Theologians have argued for ages over the problem of evil. Why does it exist? Why are people not aware of truth? These questions have been answered by the rare and gifted ones who have transcended human consciousness, with its belief in good and evil. For those who are on the plane of relative consciousness, the problem of how evil exists arises through academic and theological concepts, but saints and sages who have attained Christ consciousness tell us that evil does not exist at all. They say that we need only to know how to remove our ignorance to find that evil resides only in our sense of ego. Ego veils our eyes, and ignorance results. In reality, we are spirit. We have body, senses, and mind, but when we forget that we are spirit and identify ourselves with the body, senses, and mind, the sense of ego intervenes, and we forget our super-conscious nature. Thus, by living on the sense plane, we become subject to believing in the devil, for with our consciousness fragmented by the attractions of the sense level, we fail to understand the incompatibility of affirming the existence of both God and the devil.

So ego is the second concept one must understand, and whether one is Hindu, Buddhist, or Christian the problem of life amounts to this: How can one get rid of the ego? The answer given by the great sages of all religions is one and the same: Surrender yourself to God, and love God with all your heart, mind, and soul; let individual consciousness be absorbed by God consciousness. It sounds so simple to get rid of the ego, but it is the most difficult thing one can possibly do. If right discipline, patience, and perseverance are practiced, it is possible. But the mind's tendencies toward the pleasant are usually stronger than its tendencies toward the good, and the ego perpetually reasserts itself. Continuous sincere effort is therefore the only way to get rid of it.

The third concept is belief. We often console ourselves with the thought that God is sufficient for enlightenment, but unless there is a clear conception of what this means, unfoldment cannot occur. Distorted beliefs halt growth; knowledge alone dispels the darkness of ignorance. Believing in God is a positive help, but enlightenment is not possible without direct experience. No freedom is possible through mere belief—in order to gain freedom, one must have an earnest desire to attain higher knowledge.

A one-pointed mind is essential to God realization. We should approach truth through one way only. If one practices meditation in one way today and another tomorrow, for instance, it does not make the mind one-pointed. Some teachers give their students many different objects to meditate upon, but this does not help the mind to become steady. Unless there is only one chosen ideal or object to love or meditate upon, there cannot be any progress. Single-minded devotion toward one's ideal is very important. If one's ideal is Christ, then it is helpful to know that this same ideal is the absolute unmanifested One who is meditated upon by others in various names and forms. The Christ is your soul, and you should learn to see him in all beings, to feel and know that he is your shepherd and treasure. You should awaken the faculty of spiritual discrimination to know the difference between the real and the unreal. Then you will know that Christ is the abiding Reality and that all else is merely appearance. With such knowledge, liberation is possible, but it should be combined with earnest desire, sincere effort, and spiritual discipline. Otherwise, progress is impossible.

Prayer is the fourth concept to be understood. It is communication between the lower and higher domains, and it often takes the shape of a petition. Many people mistake prayer for meditation, which is the continuation of one thought. In meditation, individual interests are transcended by a one-pointed mind that desires to fathom the desireless and unfathomable realms of life. There is a further difference between petitionary prayer and meditation: in petitionary prayer there is always a demand for something, but in meditation one transcends the thinking process and all conditioning of the mind. Prayer is also different from contemplation, in which one ponders certain ideals. Prayer and contemplation are dualistic, but in meditation, when the final state has been reached, there is a direct "yoking" of the soul with God, and a monistic state is realized. All metaphysical and religious laws are left behind when one reaches this highest state of unity, and only meditation expands individual consciousness to universal Christ consciousness.

The Unfoldment of Meditation

The word *meditation* is used in various ways, but however it is used, it always refers to techniques that deal with one's inner nature. Through these techniques one finally transcends all levels of the mind and goes on to Christ consciousness and realization of the absolute One. Meditation does not require a belief in dogma or in any authority. It is an inward journey in which one studies one's own self on all levels, and ultimately reaches the source of consciousness. The aim of meditation is Self-realization—a direct vision of Truth. It is not an intellectual pursuit, nor is it emotional rapture. One's whole being is involved. It is neither suppression, which makes one passive, nor is it the acquisition of any experience that is not already within us. Meditation leads one from want to wantlessness. It is a way of going from the known to the unknown. The process can hardly be explained by words, but it leads one from the personal, through the transpersonal, and finally unites one with the highest One. It transforms the whole personality.

Life is a series of experiences, but all experiences do not lead us and become guides in the path of unfoldment. There are experiences, however, that great sages have witnessed from the deeper realms of their being—experiences that do not come from the contact of the senses with sense objects. The sages talk of the bliss that proceeds from the inner depths of the self, the eternal spring of bliss that lies within the heart of man. Realization of this bliss brings life-fulfillment and wisdom. Like the kingdom of heaven in the parable of Jesus, it is found not in some place remote from life, but within life itself:

> And when he was demanded of the Pharisees, when the kingdom of God should come, he answered them and said, The kingdom of God cometh not with observation. Neither shall they say, Lo, here! or, Lo, there! for, behold, the kingdom of God is within you. (Luke 17:20-21)

By what means can such an experience be obtained? Frequently, Western Christians condemn the philosophy of meditation, but it is actually the heart of Christianity. Yoking with God, or Christ consciousness, cannot be realized by merely reciting the verses of the Bible or the sayings of Christ.

> Man, if thou wishest to know what it is to pray ceaselessly: Enter into thyself, and interrogate the Spirit of God. (Angelus Silesius Cherub 1:237)

Jesus expresses this truth in the New Testament:

> Ask, and it shall be given unto you; seek and ye shall find; knock, and it shall be opened unto you. For every one that asketh, receiveth; and he that seeketh, findeth; and to him that knocketh, it shall be opened. (Matt. 7:7-8)

> And when thou prayest, thou shalt not be as the hypocrites are: for they love to pray standing in the synagogues and in the corners of the streets, that they may be seen of men. Verily I say unto you, they have their reward. But thou, when thou prayest, enter into thy closet, and when thou has shut thy door, pray to thy Father which is in secret; and thy Father which seeth in secret shall reward thee openly. (Matt. 6:5-6)

Jesus said, "Seek and ye shall find," but how do we realize this truth? When one forgets his true nature, that "kingdom of God within," he loses his way in the tangle of the world. Who will show him the way back to what he has forgotten? Only he himself can do this. The purer the mind, the more easily it is controlled and disciplined, and a pure, disciplined mind finds its way to God. The whole process of spiritual and ethical discipline leads one to the awareness of the reality existing behind personality and nature. Through the senses one becomes aware of differences, but through Christ consciousness one becomes aware of the unity that is behind these differences. Just as ethics discovers laws that link the different aspects of sense experience, the philosophy of meditation unravels the laws of yoking the individual with the ultimate One.

Meditation is a search within oneself on various levels that finally leads one to that center from whence consciousness flows. A proper method of meditation helps one to discover the ultimate unifying principle of the universe. When methods for spiritual growth are properly understood and rightly practiced they will guide one toward the only way of transcending the self and going to the superconscious state.

In other words, when one is moved by the deeper problems and starts questioning oneself, mere promises in the scriptures are not satisfying. When one realizes the importance of life and its purpose, then one turns to the philosophy of meditation and finds the solutions therein. Patanjali, for instance, in the Yoga Sutras, outlines a systematic and detailed training program that is free of religious bias. The millions of people in both the East and the West who are genuinely interested in meditation can follow his guidelines regardless of their religion.

From the very beginning, meditation requires a seeking, questioning, and logical mind, aided by the help of the right method. In addition, the seeker must perform actions selflessly, with love, one-pointedness, self-purity, and righteousness. Otherwise, the yoking of the mind is not possible. Thus, can meditation, in its creative and dynamic aspects, be practiced. But first one must develop by having the right spiritual attitude by performing selfless action in the external world. This is called meditation in action. Another method of meditation is to sit in a calm and quiet place, on a firm seat, in a relaxed and comfortable posture, and then become aware of the breath and make the mind one-pointed by allowing it to attend to the flow of breath. When the mind has become concentrated, the *mantra* (a sound or word to make the mind one-pointed) given for meditation should be remembered. Constant remembrance of the mantra leads the student to a higher state of mind, and such a mind is capable of going beyond its limitations. Finally, when the mind goes beyond the dimensions of its own created conditions, there dawns Christ consciousness.

This second type of meditation has been practiced by yogis and monks who have devoted their whole lives to realizing the Truth. First, they withdraw their sense awareness from the objects of the world and their physical selves. Second, they concentrate the mind on a mantra, and then, when the mind starts flowing like a stream of oil, it becomes one-pointed and can transcend the

the mind on a mantra, and then, when the mind starts flowing like a stream of oil, it becomes one-pointed and can transcend the limitations of emotional and rational boundaries. Thus new habits are formed and old habits are cast off. This is called spiritual rebirth. In other words, when the mind constantly thinks of God, meditation becomes a constant remembrance, and it flows like an unbroken stream. In such a case there cannot be any bondage. Constant recollection and ceaseless prayer become a means to liberation, and meditation becomes constant remembering. So in order to have an unbroken memory of God, one should meditate regularly. The mind should flow unceasingly toward God within. Then, when one constantly lives, moves, and has his being in God, the body becomes a temple.

Theology says that God exists and that we should believe in Him. Philosophy says that we should know the relationship between the individual, the universe, and the Creator. Meditation gives a direct vision of God in the temple of the body. A meditator does not have to search, roam, or wander in pursuit of God; a meditator finds the beloved within. The foolish person keeps searching on the sense plane, for all the distractions are at the outer gate of the temple. But when one enters into the inner chamber, shutting the outer gate, one finds his majesty, the center of Christ consciousness. Then one is reborn and becomes a free citizen of the kingdom of God. Such a person becomes universal. The practice of love is the natural awareness of God, and those who are constantly aware of the reality of the Lord within become the beloved of the Lord. They alone gain liberation; they receive direction and can guide others.

Thus, to be perfect and to attain the kingdom of heaven is the attainable goal of humankind. It is within us all. We stand midway between the visible and invisible worlds—but to get to the inner experience we must abstract ourselves from the outer. It should be remembered that all great religions teach the same fundamental truth, but that the great messengers of this truth tear down traditional values and establish a new order, according to the needs of their times. That is what Erasmus meant when he delivered the great dictum, "Wherever you encounter truth, look upon it as Christianity." By transcending national, religious, and traditional boundaries, meditation transforms an individual into a cosmic person. The result of meditation is therefore revolution, for it brings about the transformation of the personality of the meditator. False values are left behind and new values are established. Thus starts reformation in the world.

Energy of Consciousness in the Human Personality

From Metaphors of Consciousness *(1981)*

The universe is a dance of energies that vibrate at many frequencies. They ebb and flow, merge and part, form ripples, tides, currents, eddies, and whirlpools. They become units of all sizes, from atoms to stars, from individual souls to cosmic beings, and again they dissolve into each other. As rays, streaks, streams, rivers, oceans of light, they flow into each other and separate again, changing frequencies—and in changing frequencies, they become suns, galaxies, spaces, airs, winds, fires, liquids, solids. They become the bodies of human beings into which the energy called consciousness comes and is embodied.

Of all the flowing energies in the universe, consciousness is the most dominant, the one from which all the others proceed and into which they all merge. The ancient texts are fond of the phrase, "from consciousness down to the solid earth," for all this is a single matrix, a tantra of energy, and within it are myriads of matrices, woven and interwoven. The human being is one such matrix of energies—ebbing, flowing, dancing at frequencies ranging from those of solid bones all the way to the subtlest waves of consciousness. Those who can understand this personality matrix will understand the whole universe.

Observe the creation of a single human personality. As two human streams of consciousness love each other, the force of their love invites a third one for whom they provide a minute body. This third one brings along in its wake a matrix of energy, and its body

197

grows along the lines of this energy. The fetus is connected to the mother at the navel, and it is from the navel that seventy-two thousand energy channels, or *nadis* in Sanskrit, fan out into the personality system. Since the energy pattern is arranged in a symmetrical manner, the body grows in a beautifully symmetrical way. For instance, look at even the hairlines of the body, and you can see how they are patterned along the symmetrical paths of the energy flow.

The personality of the fetus or of a fully grown human being is not separate from the universal dance of energies. Observe how many forces interact with the biosphere, how many energies enter into it and emerge from it unceasingly. Observe how the body clock responds to solar, lunar, and stellar times, and how the blood responds to the tides in the oceans. Although all these times, tides, and forces often seem to operate individually, each answering to its own constituent rhythm, their patterns are all vibrant subsystems within the single master system of consciousness, whose dance it all is.

The vast, all-pervading oceanic energy of consciousness barely touches us with its outer fringes, and we come alive, becoming persons. The vibration frequencies in us that are too solid, too dense, not subtle enough to flow in consonance with consciousness, become our material body, the non-*I*. Energy thus condensed becomes a cell. The cell is filled with the vital energy called *prana,* which is maneuvered by the mind-energy. The *I* in us is pure consciousness. It owns and operates the body-vehicle, and it guides the mind. It is the purest, finest vibrating energy.

The Matrix of Life

Thus, like the rest of the universe, we are layer upon layer of energy or light, which form complex patterns in which the subtler layers are aware of the grosser ones but not vice versa (which is why they are hierarchical). Through the process of meditation and self-awareness, however, it is possible for us to attune ourselves to these energy processes. In fact, all of our information in this regard comes to us from the experiences imparted through the oral tradition by great meditation masters. Others who follow this path of self-awareness will eventually know the dance that the personality, and the universe, and all the energies flowing between and within them, are dancing. There is no greater excitement than that of suddenly discovering that the universal ocean of prana is flowing right through us, that our brains are but so many stepping areas in the great dance of the universal mind, and that all that I claim to be is simply a "thrill" passing into this person *I* from the universal consciousness. And then the single point of this dynamic thrill becomes diffuse, and its millions of sparks, like an incredible display of fireworks, rush out into a vast network of energy channels that are spread throughout my person, to vitalize me, to make me mentally and physically a living being, to illuminate me so that I can say "I."

Those whose awareness is bound to the earthly level frequencies know, as the real person, only the physical body. Others, who refine their self-identification by attuning to finer frequencies, know of an undying consciousness. To know this is to know that we are immortal. But before we can reach the point of comprehending the immortality of our universal consciousness, it is essential that we understand the relationships between and among various hierarchical levels of energy. This understanding is not an intellectual process. It is a matter of letting our interior awareness travel along the lines of diffuse patterns of energy so that we can actually perceive all their modes of power and its operation. The yogi does this. He sends his awareness on this incredible interior journey and returns from it to chart for others the maps of consciousness. There is no other way to comprehend what consciousness is, what roles it plays in running our personalities.

The yogi finds that the energies (of various levels of subtlety ranging from the low frequency, earthly, solid manifestation to the very high frequency, almost undetectable mental waves) all interact with each other in many forms; he finds that the relationship between the denser and finer energies is that of interdependence. The denser ones affect the finer ones in a more immediate way, but the finer ones turn out to be the masters in the long run. Take, for example, our dense body. Its bad posture adversely affects the flow of breath, but when the will in our consciousness decides that the breath be made to flow perfectly, the body has to arrange itself in a posture that will facilitate the flow.

The relationship between the body and prana may be viewed similarly. A bad posture clogs the pathways of prana. But it is the experience of those who practice the subtler varieties of hatha yoga that once the blocks on the prana's pathways have been removed through the practice of postures, the prana itself begins to give little surges into the organs so that the body rights itself inadvertently into correct posture. What is more, many practitioners of kundalini yoga report that as a result of their practices, an involuntary cleansing of internal systems takes place, which affects the prana matrix and thereby influences the body.

The relationship between prana and mind energies is no different. An incidence of low prana may befog the mind for the time being. But again, the will of consciousness infuses the mind with a certain illumination, and then prana has no alternative but to obey the mind. Thus, through deep meditation, the mind can be used to intensify the strength of prana.

As we have hinted above, the key to the relationship between the various energies is the will that is inherent in consciousness. *Will*, however, should not be confused with the much-used term *will power*, which has become a word that almost connotes violence. Will power is an exertion of the lower mind. Will is simply an inherent quality of consciousness through which consciousness directs all its operations. These operations then affect our exterior environment and become our actions. One who cultivates self-awareness observes and, through the will, consciously controls all the interior operations of mind, prana, and body.

The higher-frequency energies contain within themselves all the power of the lower frequencies, but not vice versa (again, they are hierarchical in nature). By the same token, the mind can measure all the powers of the body and senses, but they in turn cannot measure much of the mind's power. It is for this reason that some modern scientific instruments can measure physiological signs of a certain mental state but are powerless to measure the state itself. In other words, one may measure delta brain waves, but a "depth gauge" to measure the experience of sleep itself has not as yet been invented.

This leads us to some very interesting observations about the mental state of sleep. An examination of the body, of course, reveals that one is asleep. The question then arises as to whether the signs seen in the body can tell us everything about the mental state of sleep. The answer, certainly, is no. The yogis say that only a certain surface of the mind is asleep but that a vast area of the mind never sleeps. For if the entire mind were to sleep, who is it that would continue the digestive processes during that time? Who would keep the lungs breathing and the heart pumping? If the entire mind were to sleep, who would wake us up again? Seeing that the body (which is run by the mind) maintains some of its operations during sleep, we surmise that a part of the mind must remain awake; but if we simply depend on body consciousness to experience that mind which remains awake while we sleep, we are left helpless. Yet we know that the will of consciousness is operant in the mind in order to keep the body functioning and to wake us up again. Thus it becomes clear that the finer energies cannot be contained in, or measured by, the denser ones, but the opposite is not the case.

Levels of Self-identification

Our greatest concern in a study of the relationship among energies within the human personality is with the question of self-identification, called *abhimana* in Sanskrit. In the average individual, consciousness has gravitated to identification with the densest energy level, the body—or so it appears. But, in fact, consciousness can identify with each of the forms the energy takes and call them all *I*. For instance, a person may identify his relationships with various members of his family. Consider these four statements: "He is my father, I am his son; she is my sister, I am her brother; she is my wife, I am her husband; she is my daughter, I am her father." In each statement, the *I* is common, but the relationship differs. The person saying "I" has the experience of being in all four roles—those of son, brother, husband, and father. But each of his relatives can play only a single role with him. The wife cannot know him as a son, the sister cannot identify with the "father" role in him. Yet he is all four states within himself. He is also apart from these—just himself—when sitting and writing a poem to his divine lover. He is free of all human relationships at that time, yet he is even closer to his true identity. It is thus with consciousness. At the level of the body we identify consciousness with the body and it says, "Yes, body too is made of my being, but I also breathe in breath, animate the body through prana, and think when I am mind. And yet I dwell in my own nature apart from these at all times. They are my modes, but I am not their mode. They are my variations, but I am the theme."

In other words, even though most human beings seem to identify with only the surfaces of their bodies, consciousness remains wide awake and active elsewhere too, for if their identifications were truly limited to the surfaces of their bodies (as in the case of someone sleeping), how could they breathe with the lungs, digest with the internal organs, and send out brain waves? On a still deeper level, how could they have internal emotions and other forms of thought? Obviously, consciousness is operant in and identified with each of these forms of energy even though it appears that their main identification is with the surface of the body. As we cultivate meditative self-awareness, we gradually proceed from the exterior to the interior self-identification of consciousness—first with the body, then the prana, then many stages of mind, one after another, and finally, with *pure* consciousness alone.

A question is often asked, "How did consciousness ever lose its purity in the first place?" The answer is that it never did. Just as one's whole mind is never asleep even though the sleeping part does not know of the ever-awake part, and just as a person's sister does not know him as his daughter's father, so identification with body consciousness is vastly different from identification with pure consciousness, or the One. But the full and pure consciousness continues on, taking care of all its children—the lower-level frequencies that are powerless to contain and measure it.

Regarding this question of the purity of consciousness, the ancient texts on the nature of consciousness have repeatedly made this assertion: "Who are you that asks this question?" A being identifying yourself with the consciousness as it extends into the body? Just move a bit on the spectrum. Keep moving. All of those colors reflect the same light. When did light ever cease to be light? The green is green and the red is red, but the light is always light. Only when you identify the light with one of its modes do you see blue or red. See all of consciousness, and your body is included.

Are there special procedures, processes, or connections that consciousness follows in running our personalities? The universal consciousness principle may be compared, for our purpose here, to a current into which, through many sockets, various electric appliances are plugged. The same one current supplies cooling power to the cooler, heating power to the heater, helps a radio to tune into sound waves, and the TV to gather and project visual images. So also is the consciousness principle (the primary force from which all other energies are derived) connected into all living beings, supplying to each its/his/her power for will, knowledge, and action.

Centers of Consciousness

In human beings this primary consciousness becomes operative through a system of psychophysiological centers. So far we have been traveling along the finest current. Now we begin to look from the opposite, grosser end called the physical body. This body with all its cells, as we said earlier, is run by prana; the prana is directed by the mind and the mind is guided by consciousness. There are areas in our human personality where these various energies are joined together in close consonance, resonating to each other's vibrations, deriving their power from consciousness, which, however, is absolute in itself and resonates to no other. In these specific areas the vibration passes from consciousness into the mind-prana-body system—and from these areas the energy is distributed into the rest of the personality. These are the psychophysiological centers that are plugged into the current of consciousness and that respond to its universal rhythm.

Take, for example, our breathing process. What is the origin of breath which, when looked at physically, is nothing but a series of pockets of air trapped into certain cavities? What turns that air into flowing breath? The rhythm of the movement of certain organs. What moves the organs? The prana. What causes the prana to vibrate so that the organs linked to its specific areas should thus move rhythmically? The mind, of course. The mind is moved by consciousness.

Again, look at it differently. The universal consciousness, which makes the world dance by its power, sends the tiniest spark of its thrill through the mind into our psychophysiological centers in such locations as the navel, cardiac center, throat, and the pineal area. The thrill creates a pulsation in the prana system that in turn creates certain rhythmic movements in the organs connected therewith. The rhythm is synchronized, coordinated, because it originates in the same single original thrill. Through this process, air, which would otherwise remain trapped in the cavities (as in a dead body) begins to flow as a smooth stream, and we say that the child has begun to breathe. On the other hand, when the thrill of consciousness is withdrawn, the breath simply becomes trapped air, and the doctor says that the person is dead. He who understands the source of the thrill knows that the rhythm of his breath responds to the same vibration that produces pulsations in the hearts of suns. It is thus that the yogis give to some of their breathing exercises names such as "piercing through the sun," *surya-vedhana.*

We need to further elaborate as to how consciousness becomes operative in the personality. It is not subject to limitations of space, time, dimensions, or personalities in its full universal identification. It is sent forth into our being, which is made of lower and denser frequencies, like a straight beam of light penetrating through a rocky cave. Because the lower-frequency energies vibrate in a time-space reference, creating a physical body, a physical locus has to be assumed in us for that light which transcends all loci. So the yogis say that this immense, intense energy beam of consciousness, the kundalini, is located in us in a channel extending from the base of the spine up to and engulfing the entire brain region. Though nonphysical (and therefore not tangible), it is experienced by the yogis in deep meditation as an unceasing flash of rod-like lightning shining with a light like that of ten thousand suns, yet as slim as though it were a ten-thousandth of a hair's breath in width. It passes through seven ever-vibrant and dynamic psychophysiological stations or centers into which it sends its sparks, whereby they become functional and the personality becomes operant. Thus the consciousness touches us and we come alive, becoming persons.

It is not difficult to locate these centers of consciousness or chakras. They are all marked in one way or another. Their locations are: (1) the base of the spine and the perineum, (2) the root of the genitals, (3) the navel, (4) the cardiac region between the breasts, (5) the hollow of the throat, (6) between the eyebrows, and (7) the top of the head.

Many times it is asked if the consciousness and the energy of these centers or chakras flow in the spine or in the front of the body. The answer is that the distinction is arbitrary and imaginary. The front and back locations exist only with reference to the materially dense body, but the field of finer energies permeates the entire region and does not correspond to the dimensions that are assumed with reference to the spaces and times to which the body is bound.

Tuning to the Higher Levels

The consciousness that has descended into us as the kundalini contains in it both life and awareness. It may be called the life force *(jiva-shakti)* or the consciousness force *(chit-shakti)*. Through the chakras, a division of its two powers occurs, for in order for the personality to function, a certain specialization becomes necessary. A semblance of awareness is imparted to the energy called the mind, and at the same time aliveness and vitality of the cells, organs, and senses also comes into operation through prana receiving the infusion of life energy from the kundalini. Thus the two powers of the kundalini consciousness devolve onto the mind and prana, and through them they are further infused into the entire personality. The thrill of life and awareness, however, that passes through the psychophysiological stations into the personality, is so minute compared to the actual power of consciousness, that yogis repeatedly tell us that the true consciousness is lying dormant, asleep in us.

All that humankind has ever accomplished or created, all that ever passes through an individual human being, is no more than a minute fraction of the universal consciousness. But the majority of human beings are not capable of experiencing even this minute thrill at its fullest, because the lower-level energies are not capable of containing or measuring higher-level energies. By the same token, if given more than the requisite voltage, any energy system will overload and blow up the circuits. We have established such strong identification with lower-level energies (the body, emotions, etc.) that we have weakened our power system and made it incapable of receiving a larger dose of the thrill. So we have to purify the personal consciousness and gradually tune it to its higher-level energies until enough strength is built up in the system for us to be able to awaken to the full glory that is flowing into us even as we read this. Those who have tried experimenting with the kundalini consciousness without such preliminary purification and without expert guidance have only suffered damage to both the psyche and the body.

In us, the gates of the chakras are thus open only enough to permit a mild infusion of consciousness. But look at the intense awareness we have in these centers. Even that mild infusion of dormant energy leaves us restless in each center. Look at what goes on in us at each of these stations: in the perineum and the genital areas, the sensations can sometimes seem to be uncontrollable; in the navel region, the hungers cannot be satiated; the pull of rising emotions felt in the cardiac region keeps thousands of psychiatrists busy; and all the words that we have ever spoken from the larynx are not quite enough. As to the forehead and the brain—they are the devil's very workshop. The energy already disposed through each of these centers often seems to be excessive to us, and we then say, "I just don't know what to do with my restlessness." This feeling of overload, that we are about to blow a fuse, is a common experience. It happens because the lower-frequency energies (such as those involved in ordinary physical and sense experiences) do not have the capacity to absorb all the power that is being infused into us from consciousness.

The Inward Path

The yogi resorts to a different path—the inward one. And here we come to the difference between closed stations and open stations. It is stated in the kundalini literature that an average person is living with closed chakras that are waiting to be opened. Many who are not initiated into this science erroneously think that with the opening of a chakra the outward activity in that center of consciousness will increase, thus making, let us say, a sexy person yet sexier, or an articulate person voluble! But such externalized activity only dissipates the energy at its lowest frequencies. It has nothing to do with highly refined interior consciousness.

The pulsations that we experience in ordinary daily life in the various psychophysiological stations are nothing but reminders of a higher presence within. They are like lighthouses guiding ships. Each pulsation says to our lower-level energy consciousness: "Come, this way; here is a gate through which you enter inward into the highest awareness." It leads to the place from which this minute light is sent forth. If we observe each pulsation in our personality as such a reminder, we begin to listen to an inner music, and we may use each such pulsation first as a point of focus, and then as a thread leading inward. For example, let us consider the sexual thrill in the second station. It makes an average person restless, for the infusion of energy from within is so powerful (even though it is infinitesimal compared to all the power of consciousness) that no amount of sexual activity can bring total satiety. The yogi, however, regards this center only as a gateway to higher-level energy consciousness. Its pulsations he sees only as reminders of the inner sources. He closes the outward flow, and that is called opening the chakra. All externalized restlessness then ceases. The lower-frequency energy is returned to the higher-frequency.

In other words, any time a sexual pulsation is felt in a yogi's person, he responds to it, considers it a blessing as a reminder, and uses it as the end of a thread leading inward to pure consciousness. He reverses the flow. Compared to the ecstasy of this inward flow of the personal consciousness into the universal consciousness, the outward sexual flow is a useless discharge, and all of its intense enjoyment is like sucking on the peel of an orange after squeezing out and, alas, throwing away the juice. Again, when the throat center begins to open, the yogi seeks silence. When he does utter a word it is so power-packed as to be recorded as sacred scripture and repeated for millennia around the globe. Such were the words uttered by the Buddhas and Christs of history.

We may divide human beings into those of the inward-flowing consciousness *(antar-vritti)* and those of the outward-flowing consciousness *(bahir-vritti)*. Those in the first category live and walk in the awareness of their cosmic connection. They are unceasingly and interminably conscious of the thrill of the universal divine consciousness running through them. They do not utilize any of their energies as mere persons, but serve as channels for the cosmic flow. They are dependent on nothing external and on no person, but many are dependent on them for succor, solace, knowledge, and healing. Those in the second category are those who believe that only the information passing through the senses and into the brain constitutes personality and consciousness. Their excitements are derived not from the inner thrill, but from the contact that dense senses make with yet denser exterior objects. Thus their psychology is that of a dependent person, however much they may clamor for individual freedom and claim self-dependence. Those in the first category, the rare few in the history of mankind, are committed to turning sensory awareness inward in order to free themselves from the bondage of dependence on the limited exterior and to experience the unlimited flow of cosmic energies that are at their disposal.

We need to understand how this is accomplished, how the outward flow of awareness may be reversed so that the intricate dance of the interior energies may become real. We need to understand that through the application of will we can cultivate a resolve to change our self-identification from lower-frequency energies to the higher one. That is immortality. That is freedom of consciousness from the bonds of space, time, karma, and causation. It is the dance of the freedom of energies.

The Awakening of Kundalini

From Kundalini, Evolution and Consciousness *(1979)*

The science of kundalini is one of the most advanced and difficult branches of yoga. In this article I hope to set right some misconceptions and abuses of this science and to give a clearer conception of what kundalini yoga is.

To understand the meaning of this word *kundalini* we must consider it in its proper context along with the word *Shakti,* for the term kundalini modifies and explains this term shakti. Kundalini comes from the word *kundala,* which means coiled. The image of a serpent coiled up while resting conveys the idea of kundalini. The word Shakti comes from the root *shak,* meaning to have power or to be able. Taken together, these two Sanskrit words might be translated as the coiled-up power, or the resting potential.

But what is this power and why is it resting? To understand this, we must go to the very foundation of tantric philosophy. According to this ancient philosophy, the entire universe is a manifestation of pure consciousness. In manifesting the universe, this pure consciousness seems to become divided into two poles or aspects, neither of which can exist without the other. One aspect retains a static quality and remains identified with unmanifest consciousness. In tantra this quality is called *Shiva* and is conceptualized as masculine. Shiva is depicted as being absorbed in the deepest state of meditation, a state of formless Being, Consciousness, and Bliss. He remains for the most part aloof and is uninterested in manifesting the universe. Shiva has the power to be, but not the power to become or change. He has no power to act

211

or to manifest. He is the power holder but has no energy in his own right. Nevertheless, consciousness as the power that builds the world is based on and arises out of this consciousness as being.

The other part of this polarity is a dynamic, energetic, or creative aspect that is called Shakti, the great mother of the universe, for it is from her that all form is born. Shakti is the subtlest of created things. She manifests herself as the entire universe including matter, life, and mind.

These two principles are united, but in the manifest world an illusion of separation is created between pure consciousness and its manifestations. Shakti is a projection of consciousness that veils the consciousness from which she was projected. The innumerable illusory manifestations (*maya*) that she brings forth are called the universe. The scriptures say that when karma ripens, Shakti "becomes desirous of creation, and covers herself with her own maya."[1] The creation of this illusion is called *involution,* for we find consciousness *involving* or folding over upon itself. As a result of this involvement it seems to become complex, bipolar, and formed. After aeons of time, when the universe is dissolved, it is drawn or recollected into that Shakti that produced it. This latter process is known as *evolution.* It is a further state of development in which consciousness becomes uninvolved with its manifestation.

We know from physics that energy exists in two forms: (1) dynamic or active and (2) latent or potential, power at rest. Any activity or force must have a static background. When consciousness manifests itself as the creative or dynamic principle (Shakti), Shakti then in turn polarizes herself into these two forms also. In the manifestation of the universe, part of the energy of Shakti becomes involved in the manifestation itself, while a still greater part remains dormant. The dynamic aspect is Shakti in specific differentiated form. In Indian mythology the primal power, that which remains latent after the ongong creation is manifested, is symbolized by coiled-up energy in the form of a serpent that supports the universe.

Organization of Energies in the Human Body

According to tantra, the human being is a minature universe. All that is found in the cosmos can be found within each individual, and the same principles that apply to the universe apply in the case of the individual being. In human beings the surplus of energy that is not being used to maintain the functioning of the organism is also symbolically described as a coiled or resting serpent. This potential energy is said to rest at the base of the spinal cord, at the *muladhara* (root support) chakra. The potential energy is called kundalini. Kundalini is the static support of the entire body and all of its pranic or energy forces. "Kundalini Shakti in individual bodies is . . . the *static center* around which every form of existence as moving power revolves."[2] "Kundalini is the Divine Cosmic Energy in bodies."[3]

The dynamic energy that provides the working forces for the body evolves from the active energy of Shakti and is called *prana.* Electrical energy is more subtle than mechanical energy. Its properties have come to be recognized and utlized in the past two hundred to three hundred years. Before that the idea of electrical forces was quite foreign to the thinking of most people. This is the situation today with our empirical understanding of prana. Prana is a still more subtle form of energy that is not yet studied or understood in the mainstream of modern science. However, it has been studied in detail in the introspective sciences of yoga.

Prana is organized and subdivided according to specific functions in the body. It flows like an electric current through an intricate network of subtle nerves (*nadis*), connecting the body and mind and keeping the entire organism in working order. This vital force of Shakti in the body is also organized around specific centers. These are not physical centers, although they have physical correspondences in the various plexuses of the body. These energy centers, called *chakras,* are intricate vortices of energy that help organize the physical body, although they cannot be perceived by it. The chakras influence, vitalize, and control corresponding regions of the body. They also determine the quality of consciousness. When the universal consciousness is manifest in the form of each center, the result is a particular frame of reference through which the individual experiences the world. For example, when mind and energy are expressed through the *svadhishthana* chakra, one may be preoccupied with sensual enjoyment, while at another, the *anahata* chakra, one becomes loving and compassionate, interested in taking care of others. As Table 1 indicates, each of these centers in the individual has its own corresponding *loka* or cosmic plane of reality. In other words, there are realms (in Western terminology, earthly, celestial, or heavenly spheres) in which the mode of experience corresponds to that of each chakra.

TABLE 1

No.	Psychic Center in the Human Body	Corresponding Physical Center	Loka or Cosmic Plane	Guna or Quality
6	Ajna	Pituitary	Satyaloka	Sattva
5	Vishuddha	Thoraxic Plexus	Tapaloka	Sattva
4	Anahata	Cardiac Plexus	Janoloka	Rajas
3	Manipura	Solar Plexus	Maharloka	Rajas
2	Svadhisthana	Sacral Plexus	Survarloka	Tamas
1	Muladhara	Coccyx	Bhuvarloka	Tamas

Although there are many energy centers, six are traditionally considered to be most important. These are located along the central axis of the body in conjunction with the spinal cord (see Figure 1). Energy is usually focused in one or more of these centers to the relative exclusion of others. Differences in where energy is focused from person to person and from time to time help to account for differences in the way the world is experienced from one individual to the next, and from one moment to the next.

The two lowest centers are grouped together because they represent the most primitive expressions of energy and states of consciousness that are most closely tied to the physical world. They are linked to the basic instincts for individual and species survival. When energy is focused in these centers, pure con-

survival. When energy is focused in these centers, pure consciousness is obscured, and the individual identifies with the grossest material plane of existence. These chakras have the quality of *tamas* (inertia or torpor).

The second two chakras, located at the solar and cardiac plexuses, represent a turning to more subtle relationships with the world. There is an active involvement in trying to organize and make sense of the world, and to interact on a less physical plane than in the case of the first two chakras. There is a focus on the building up and expansion of one's sense of I-ness. The predominant characteristic is that of *rajas* (expansion and activity).

The two chakras that correspond to the cervical and pituitary centers in the human body represent a movement away

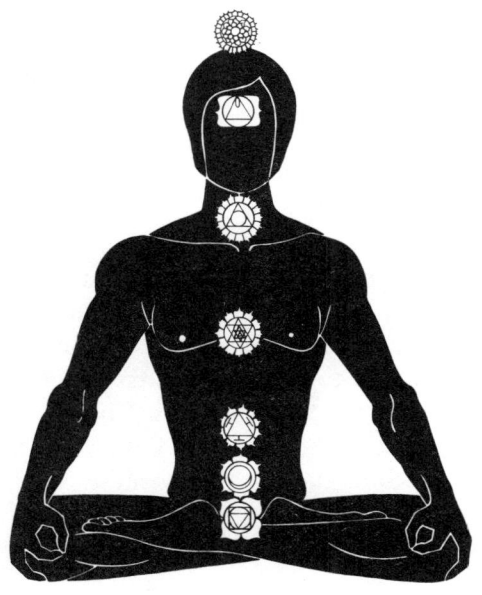

Figure 1. The chakras in traditional symbolic form.

from worldly relationships to a world of pure form. Here one perceives and relates to the underlying forms from which the material universe comes. One who is operating at these levels exhibits creativity, intuition, and wisdom. His manner is predominantly *sattvic* (serene and devotional).

There is a series of still more subtle chakras above the ajna or pituitary center, culminating in the center of pure consciousness at the crown of the head. This is the abode of Shiva, pure transcendent consciousness, in each individual. This center is named *sahasrara* (the place of luster). Its corresponding cosmic plane is called *chandra* loka (the world of nectar). Ordinarily the individual is polarized, with Shiva residing at the crown chakra and the latent power of Shakti (kundalini) lying dormant at the base of the spine. Only the smallest bit of Shakti's energy becomes dynamic and functions in the chakras and nadis (subtle nerve channels) in order to maintain the ordinary functions of the individual. That such an infinite reservoir of energy exists is not even imagined by Western science.

Activating the Latent Potential

It is traditionally thought that Shakti contains not only latent energy but also latent memories, both personal and transpersonal. The modern way of understanding this latent power is in terms of the unconscious. Like Shakti, the unconscious is conceived of as a vast unknown power. Those individuals who have controlled access to the unconscious experience an abundance of energy, insight, and creativity. So it is with the latent power of Shakti. Those who transform this force from its latent to its active form become the dynamic geniuses of every age and culture.

This transformation is called the awakening of kundalini. Usually this is depicted as a sudden, intense, earthshaking, transforming experience. But such an experience is rare. It is more usual for tiny bits of this energy to be released through various means. One then experiences breakthroughs, bursts of energy and enthusiasm, peak experiences, a sense of well-being, and similar changes in consciousness. This is analogous to what happens in psychotherapy as bits of the unconscious are brought into one's awareness. Occasionally there are more startling breakthroughs in which a significant quantity of the latent power is released. This leads to more unusual experiences, which will later be described.

The practice of kundalini yoga involves not only awakening this kundalini Shakti but also systematically leading her through each of the chakras to the sahasrara or crown chakra, the abode of Shiva. The word yoga means union, and this union can be understood as the uniting of kundalini Shakti with Shiva (pure consciousness). When this is achieved in the individual, he becomes fully conscious. There is no longer an unconscious or latent power—the individual is fully awakened and illumined. When the static Shakti becomes dynamic and travels upward, fully energizing each of the centers along the way, the polarization of the body gives way, consciousness of the body is withdrawn, and one attains the highest state of *samadhi*. Sir John Woodroffe eloquently says:

> When Kundalini Shakti *sleeps* in the Muladhara, man is *awake* to the world; when she *awakes* to unite, and does unite, with the supreme static Consciousness which is Shiva, then consciousness is *asleep* to the world and is one with the Light of all things.[4]

As a static power, kundalini sustains consciousness of the world, but when she unites with Shiva, she loses consciousness of the world and goes to a state of consciousness without object or form. When she is aroused and moves upward, kundalini withdraws into herself the dynamic forces that maintain the body. This is the reverse of involution, of consciousness involving itself in the universe. It is a process of evolution in which the human being comes to realize his full potential. The final goal of the yogi is to dissolve the universe and abide in that state of pure consciousness.

Outwardly the body may seem no longer to be alive, but it continues to function minimally so that it can again be used as an instrument of the individual who has temporarily left it. The body may even become cold as a corpse. It is said that the union of Shiva and Shakti generates a nectar that continues to sustain the body in this superconscious state.

This union is the goal of the aspirant, but few achieve it. It is more common, although still rare, for the yogi to awaken kundalini Shakti and lead her only part of the way toward the goal.

Preparaton for Awakening Kundalini

A number of methods have been developed in yoga to help the aspirant awaken the sleeping force withn. An appropriate method is chosen by a realized teacher to prepare each student according to his particular inclinations and capacities. Before decribing these mehtods, I would like to warn the student so that he may avoid being misguided by those who claim to be teachers of these practices but do not have the necessary realization to guide their students properly.

Kundalini and tantra yoga are perhaps the most misunderstood and abused of all yoga practices. These sacred, systematic, and extremely advanced traditions for leading the aspirant to the highest state of transcendent consciousness have been caricatured in the West in crude breathing exercises and in unfounded claims by a number of teachers who say that they directly arouse this energy in many of their students through their mere touch or presence. All too often what becomes aroused are the latent hysterical tendencies in the student, who imagines and acts out all sorts of things. The misinterpretation of these ancient, revered teachings has led to self-delusion of genuine awakening. Those who offer easy methods for achieving an awakened state of mind are in actuality using suggestion or trickery and are misleading their students. The vast majority of reports of awakened kundalini that we find in the West are merely the expressions of rich imaginations.

It should be no surprise that the study and practice of kundalini Shakti should be so abused. Whenever the awakening power in any form is offered, those who seek to aggrandize themselves flock to those who promise rapid and easy attainment of such power. They are finally duped by their own desire for power. All they catch is the illusion of power, never the real thing. Once I asked my master why there are so many false teachers in the world. He said, "They create a fence for those who are genuine. By attracting those students who want to get something for nothing, they free the real teacher to work with a smaller group of sincere aspirants."

To genuinely awaken kundalini, one must first prepare himself. Without long and patient practice in purifying oneself and stengthening one's capacity to tolerate and assimilate such a flood of energy, the awakening of this latent power would deeply disturb, disorient, and confuse the student. Even at the physical level such a charge of energy can threaten the integrity of the body. This has been metaphorically described in terms of the body being a ten-ampere fuse receiving a current of one hundred amperes at a high potential. Only after one has developed considerable self-control can this charge be tolerated without the organism's being strained to the point of danger.

The experience of a "bad trip" after ingesting a powerful psychoactive drug is nothing compared to the release of this force in one who is unprepared. Can you imagine the effect of the sudden and massive release into awareness of what is in your unconscious? This is exactly what happens with the awakening of the kundalini. If through careful training the aspirant has gradually come to recognize and master his unconscious demons— in other words, has purified and strengthened himself—then and only then is he prepared to face the full awakening of all that is latent within him. In Indian iconography, Shakti

> is painted as riding on a lion as a symbol of strength, magnanimity and majesty. The picture also denotes the fact that when the Kundalini is aroused in a person, She rides the lion of yoga which roars like a hungry lion in the body and begins to devour the weakness (flesh) of the yogi. The Shakti with Her numerous kinds of weapons begins to wage war on the animal

passions which . . . hinder spiritual advancement, killing them
one by one, till every one of them has been to the last
overpowered and killed.[5]

If the aspirant has not purified himself through various spiritual
practices, the war that is waged within can be especially intense,
even unbearable. Releasing kundalini without preparation is like
opening Pandora's box without having cultivated the ability to
master what emerges. For this reason the teacher who truly
represents a tradition that teaches methods to awaken kundalini
will never fully reveal these to an unprepared student, but will do
his best to prepare him. Preparation for awakening kundalini is
more important than awakening kundalini.

Methods of Awakening

Here is a brief overview of those methods traditionally used
to prepare the student and to awaken this latent force.

1. Physical means. The practice of hatha yoga, including
purifying exercises, prepares the body to tolerate the heightened
energy of kundalini. After considerable preparation, advanced
postures, energy locks and seals called *mudras* and *bandhas,* and
breathing exercises (pranayama) help to rechannel the dynamic
energy (prana) and use it to awaken the latent energy (kundalini).
Since prana regulates the functioning of body and mind, by
acquiring control of this energy the yogi is able to control the mind
and body at will. In most people prana flows outward, connecting
the mind with the senses, but when this energy is concentrated and
channeled upward through the chakras, the mind becomes
detached from the senses and the physical body and becomes
inwardly absorbed in meditation. A number of related spiritual
exercises have the effect of withdrawing energy from two subtle
nerve channels (called *ida* and *pingala*) that run along the spinal
cord, and channeling this energy through a third channel
(*sushumna*), which runs along the center of the spine. A form of
prana that normally travels upward (*prana vayu*) is brought
downward, while the normally downward flowing energy (*apana*

vayu) is brought upward so that the two merge. The union of these two pranic currents in the central channel creates intense heat. In the Upanishads they are called upper and lower *arni*. By the friction produced between them, fire is created.

> The position seems to be thus similar to a hollow tube in which a piston is working at both ends without escape of the central air, which thus becomes heated. Then the Serpent Force, Kundalini, aroused by the heat thus generated, is aroused from her potential state.[6]

Kundalini, once thereby aroused, flows upward through a channel at the center of the spine called *Brahma nadi*.

2. Concentration and Meditation. Kundalini can also be awakened by intense concentration and meditation on specific sensory nerves, such as the tip of the nose or the root of the tongue, along with concentration and meditation on specific chakras. Such concentration helps one withdraw one's consciousness from its absorption in the physical body and master the quality of energy associated with a specific chakra. Meditation on a chakra along with the repetition of a particular thought form (*mantra*) and a visualization (*yantra*) can awaken energy from kundalini and bring it to that center.

3. *Brahmacharaya.* Physical and mental celibacy is still another path that can lead from involution to evolution. Instead of discharging the vital force in the service of procreation, the yogi who follows this path learns to absorb that energy and direct it upward. The external union between male and female is forsaken; instead an internal union between the male (Shiva) and female (Shakti) principle takes place.

4. Tantra. This union is most clearly cultivated in tantra yoga, which centers on the worship of Shakti, the mother of the universe. Many people in the West think that tantra means having sexual relations. In some forms of tantra, a male-female relationship may be involved, but it is transformed from the physical plane to the sphere of energy and consciousness. The partners relate to

one another as embodiments of Shiva and Shakti rather than as two physical beings. In the more pure form of tantra, Shakti is worshipped through meditation and mantra, so that the aspirant comes into a direct and conscious relationship with the Shiva and Shakti within and unites them. It is considered that the teacher introduces *bahiyayag* (external worship) to unprepared sutdents, but those who are prepared are introduced to *antaryag* (inner worship) to make the mind inward and one-pointed. According to the Tantra Shastras there still exist three great schools of tantra: *kaula, mishra,* and *samaya.* While kaula and mishra perform certain rituals and believe in obtaining powers (*siddhis*), the samaya group does not believe in any external rituals and is considered to be the purest and highest of all.

These are just some of the practices for arousing kundalini. She can also be awakened through intense devotion. And for those who are more intellectual and philosophical, intense study of the scriptures with a competent teacher can also serve this purpose. In fact, any spiritual practice that leads to a genuine awakening and experience of transcendent states of consciousness involves an awakening of this coiled energy.

The Teacher's Guidance

The word kundalini also means a bowl of fire. In all great mystic traditions of the world there have been similar experiences of kundalini awakening. Moses was moved to take off his shoes before the burning bush; Isaiah (in the temple) and Mohammed (on the night of power, when the teachings of the Koran were revealed to him) also experienced the awakening of this force. The books of Revelation in Judaism and Christianity reveal the signs and symptoms of the awakening of kundalini. Hindu and Buddhist scriptures make up the most extensive literature on the subject. This literature emphasizes that, particularly on this path, a competent teacher is essential.

In most of the spiritual practices, the awakening of this force is not clearly conceptualized or systematically brought under the control of the aspirant. Thus the mystic may have rare, inexplicable, and uncontrolled moments of ecstacy and illumination, but he does not know how to produce these again at will. This is not the case in the systematic practice of yoga under the guidance of a teacher who himself has mastered this latent force. Indeed it is the awakened master, as the representative of a perennial tradition, who makes it possible through the practice of kundalini yoga, but sincere effort is essential. Under the close supervision of the master and through a series of initiations the student is guided toward his goal. The first initiation on this path is the imparting of a mantra, a "seed" sound to concentrate on, which represents certain aspects of this vital force. Traditionally, mantra meditation is not given as an isolated practice but is considered an early step on the path. It is practiced in conjunction with a number of coordinate spiritual exercises and mental and physical disciplines to purify and prepare the student for further steps. If the student is successful in his practice, he is guided through more difficult and intricate forms of meditation in which he becomes sensitive to the forces within and is able to channel them.

The practices may culminate in a higher initiation called *shaktipat diksha,* in which the master directly transmits his energy to the student to remove the final obstacle, awakening the sleeping serpent and leading her upward. One who is functioning on a higher level may sometimes unconsciously influence those around him in the same way that a magnet can only attract a particular metal. As a magnet influences a particular metal, such a teacher influences those who are prepared, though he might inspire many. In shaktipat the influence is conscious and extremely intense. Through a look, touch, or thought the master transmits his own power to the aspirant, who is suddenly transported into a realm of blissful divine consciousness.

This state may last for an hour or a few days. Typically the aspirant is not able to maintain the aroused state and after some period of time kundalini returns to her abode. The awakened energy becomes latent once again. But now the aspirant's faith is strengthened, for he has directly experienced the awakened state.

It is not at all like a hypnotic trance of the hysterical outpourings that parody this state. The individual is completely transformed after such an experience. He has glimpsed Divinity, and although the experience is not yet completely integrated, it continues to influence him at all levels of his being for the rest of his life. As a result of such an experience, many latent abilities are awakened. The student becomes dynamic, creative, and talented in all aspects of life. He is elevated spiritually, morally, and intellectually. But he must also guard against an inflated ego. He must work systematically, perhaps for many years, to learn how to awaken and guide that energy within and without.

This experience of shaktipat is typically not repeated many times, for it takes considerable time for the student to integrate what he has experienced. If the master does not proceed slowly and cautiously in working with the student, the student could become disoriented and unable to function in the world for a considerable period of time. There is another less widely known practice called *shakti chalana,* in which the student is led gradually, and to some extent unconsciously, through transformations in which he becomes more and more able to integrate and handle the awakening Shakti.

Fortunately, the master is not working alone when dealing with this powerful force. He has behind him the tradition of sages, which he represents. He is guided by that tradition in determining when and how to release the latent power within his close disciple. I remember my first experience of this sort. I was still quite young and had recently been initiated by my master after many years of diligent practice under his tutelage. One day he told me that a swami would come the next morning and that I was to touch him on the forehead, thereby initiating him in shaktipat diksha. I protested, saying that I had no such power to arouse the kundalini in another person. But he said to me, "Don't you know, it is not you acting. You are just the instrument of a higher power. Let that power work through you."

I was not reassured. I could not sleep that night. I remained awake, thinking, "What if I touch him and nothing happens? He will no doubt be furious with me." I tried touching my finger to various objects to see if there was some vital force passing through me, but I was aware of nothing. When morning came, I met the swami at the appointed time, still not knowing how I would fulfill the task that was given to me. I sat in meditation with him before me, and repeated certain mantras, as I was instructed by my guru. Suddenly I found my arm being raised. It was not at all under my control. I touched that swami and he remained in samadhi for several hours. I know this was not hypnosis or my imagination. When I asked my master to explain what happened, he just smiled knowingly. I find that this power is still not in my control as an individual but is guided by the tradition with which I am linked. There may be someone to whom I wish to impart this experience, but nevertheless I cannot. Yet with a few rare individuals I feel such a strong impulse that I cannot resist.

Signs and Symptoms of Kundalini

There are clear and unmistakable signs when kundalini awakens. Initially there may be involuntary jerks of the body, trembling and shaking, and an intense feeling of pleasure. One of the first and most common occurrences is the experience of intense heat as the energy is passing through a particular center. Here are typical descriptions of the experience of heat:

> I felt a burning sensation in various parts of the body and my whole body was perspiring. I had previously seen flames . . . but they were not so extremely hot as these.

> Sometmes it seemed as if a jet of molten copper, mounting up through the spine, dashed against my crown.

As kundalini awakens there is a sensation of something moving along the spine. This has been described as a feeling of frogs jumping, snakes wriggling, or ants creeping in a line from the feet to the head. As the aroused energy passes through the chakras, yoga mudras, bandhas, or breathing exercises, which are usually practiced voluntarily, may occur spontaneously and unintentionally. Kundalini acts as a spiritual guide, governing and leading the individual through various experiences.

The aspirant may have difficulty leading the energy upward. At times it may remain for a while in one of the lower chakras and return again to its resting place. There are three *granthis* (knots) through which the energy has a difficult time passing. In piercing the abdominal knot, pain or physical disorders may occur. The yogi may have to repeat the process of awakening kundalini a number of times, gradually leading her higher along her path. Specific spiritual exercises are given by the teacher to help the student overcome the obstacles encountered. It is said that bringing kundalini to the anahata chakra at the cardiac plexus is the most difficult task. At this point kundalini is said to pass from an infant state to a mature state.

As the kundalini passes through and energizes each of the chakras, particular visions and sounds are experienced at each center. The disciple passes through the corresponding lokas or cosmic planes. He will typically see a lotus-like flower at each center with its petals hanging downward. When the energy becomes more manifest in that center, the petals turn upward. The quality or force that exists at each center is seen in the form of a presiding deity. These experiences are consistent and predictable from one individual to another. Here is an example:

> Some days later the navel lotus appeared. It was similar to the lotus of the heart but its petals were slightly different. Many days later the form of Shesasayi (Vishnu sleeping on a snake) appeared. . . . From the navel of Vishnu issued forth a lotus plant, and Brahmadeva appeared to be sitting on the flower.

More advanced yogis believe that it is only when the ajna chakra at the pituitary center is reached that anything significant is achieved. Ramakrishna said, "If . . . anybody's mind reaches the spot between the eyebrows . . . he then has direct knowledge of the supreme Self and remains continually in samadhi."[7]

There are a number of lesser known centers between the ajna chakra and the sahasrara or highest center at the crown of the head:

> When mind rises up to these stages, super-visions of light in various forms such as the moon, the sun, stars . . . etc., appear to the inner vision, and sounds of bells, drums, flutes, etc., culminating in one resembling thunder, become audible.[8]

St. Teresa of Avila describes the following experience:

> The noises in my head are so loud that I am beginning to wonder what is going on. . . . My head sounds just as if it were full of brimming rivers . . . and a host of little birds seem to be whistling, not in the ears, but in the upper part of the head, where the higher part of the soul is said to be; I have held this view for a long time, for the spirit seems to move upward with great velocity.[9]

In the yogic tradition these visions are said to culminate in the union of Shiva and Shakti at the sahasrara. This is the most transcending and all-encompassing state of consciousness that can be experienced. There is nothing beyond this. The individual consciousness becomes merged with divine consciousness.

If kundalini were to remain at this center, after twenty-one days the body would no longer be maintained. Usually, however, it is not possible to maintain this state of consciousness, and kundalini returns once again to the lower chakras. Gradually, through systematic practice, the yogi learns complete mastery of this energy and is able to direct it at will, maintaining that state of consciousness that is appropriate and useful at a given time.

Control of Body and Mind

As far as my own experience goes, I was trained to study body anatomy first, and to have control over the four appetites (food, sleep, sex, and self-preservation). I was told to have a healthy body and to discipline myself in mind, action, and speech. I was asked not to allow my mind to be influenced by anyone's opinion and way of thinking. This took a long time for me to achieve.

It is not possible for an unhealthy body and a disturbed mind to tread this path properly. A healthy body and yogic mind are two necessary instruments to awaken the consciousness and lead it to its source from where the consciousness flows on various degrees and grades. I was trained to have control over bodily functions and internal states, and without that it was not possible for me to think of awakening kundalini and going to the center of consciousness.

I have met others who hallucinate or mistakenly boast of awakening this power, but I was strictly warned not to be guided by my emotions. No doubt emotion is one of the greatest powers, but it needs to be devotionally channeled. Otherwise pleasure and joy on the physical and mental planes can be mistaken for the awakening of kundalini.

I was taught to have perfect control over the unconscious activities of my mind and autonomic and central nervous system. During my intense *sadhana* I observed perfect silence with certain dietary rules. Stillness of body and mind were two important signs of my progress. I was instructed not to be guided by any hunch of so-called intuition that comes through an untrained and un-purified mind. After completing my sadhana, which included thoroughly studying all the systems of Indian philosophy, I can assure you that those experiences that ensue from irrationality and from the exhaustion of mental force through pushing, shoving, rolling and tumbling, jumping, shouting, and weeping are not signs and symptoms of kundalini.

I determined to do research in order to scientifically verify the way this force is brought under systematic control by the yogis. In experiments at the Menninger Foundation we have shown that the autonomic nervous sytem can be brought fully under control. In various experiments I have demonstrated the voluntary control of brain waves, heart rate, and skin temperature. But these are only the minor points, the preliminary self-mastery that is necessary to awaken kundalini, and that modern science is capable of observing with its instruments and methods. More research, which goes further and studies the achievement of various higher states of consciousness, can only be conducted when science finds the methods to examine and differentiate these states from one another and from ordinary consciousness.

The awakening of kundalini is a very specialized method of self-realization that can be attained only after long, intense practice. Silence and discipline of body and mind through self-effort, as well as sincerity, faithfulness, and truthfulness, are necessary requisites in the path of enlightenment. Grace dawns at a certain state of attainment. It is important to know and awaken the ascending force, kundalini. But it is equally important to be aware of this descending force called *kripa* (grace). Shaktipat is a form of grace that dawns when sincere, selfless effort is made by the student.

For sincere aspirants it is advisable to study the tantra scriptures in a traditional way, under a competent guide, and then start practicing methods for awakening of kundalini. Modern students, out of sheer enthusiasm and emotional outbursts, surrender themselves before their emotional ideals and depend completely on their guru for enlightenment. They forget that though the guru is important, he is still a means and not the end. A real guru leads his student on the path of freedom and does not propagate a personality cult. These days many gurus, instead of introducing the subject and instructing the student in the ways and methods, ask students not to do anything except to follow them— least of all to think and to cultivate the mind. Such students may have experiences on the higher levels of consciousness, but the experiences will be temporary and superficial. Direct experience through self-mastery alone enlightens the student and leads him to the final abode. The Upanishads declare that without a systematic method of meditation (*dhyana* yoga), the awakening of kundalini is not possible. The great sages experienced the union of individual consciousness with the cosmic One through meditation. Says *Shvetashvatara* Upanishad: "The great sages by practicing the method of meditation could awaken the Devatma Shakti."

Notes

1. *Kulacudamani*, 1:16-24.

2. Sir John Woodroffe, *The Serpent Power* (Madras: Ganesh & Co., 1972), p. 42.

3. Ibid., p. 2

4. Sir John Woodroffe, *Sakti and Sakta* (Madras: Ganesh & Co., 1951), p. 446.

5. Swami Vishnu Tirtha, *Devatma Shakti* (Bombay: Sri Sadhan Granthmala Prakashan Samiti, 1962), p. 126.

6. M. P. Pandit, *Kundalini Yoga* (Madras: Ganesh & Co., 1971), p. 56.

7. Swami Savadananda, *Sri Ramakrishna the Great Master* (Mylapore, Madras: Sri Ramakrishna Math, 1952), p. 366.

8. Swami Vishnu Tirtha, op. cit., p. 96.

9. St. Therese of Avila, *Interior Castle,* tr. and ed. E. Allison Peers (Garden City, N.Y.: Doubleday & Company, Inc., 1961), pp. 77-78.

Miscellaneous

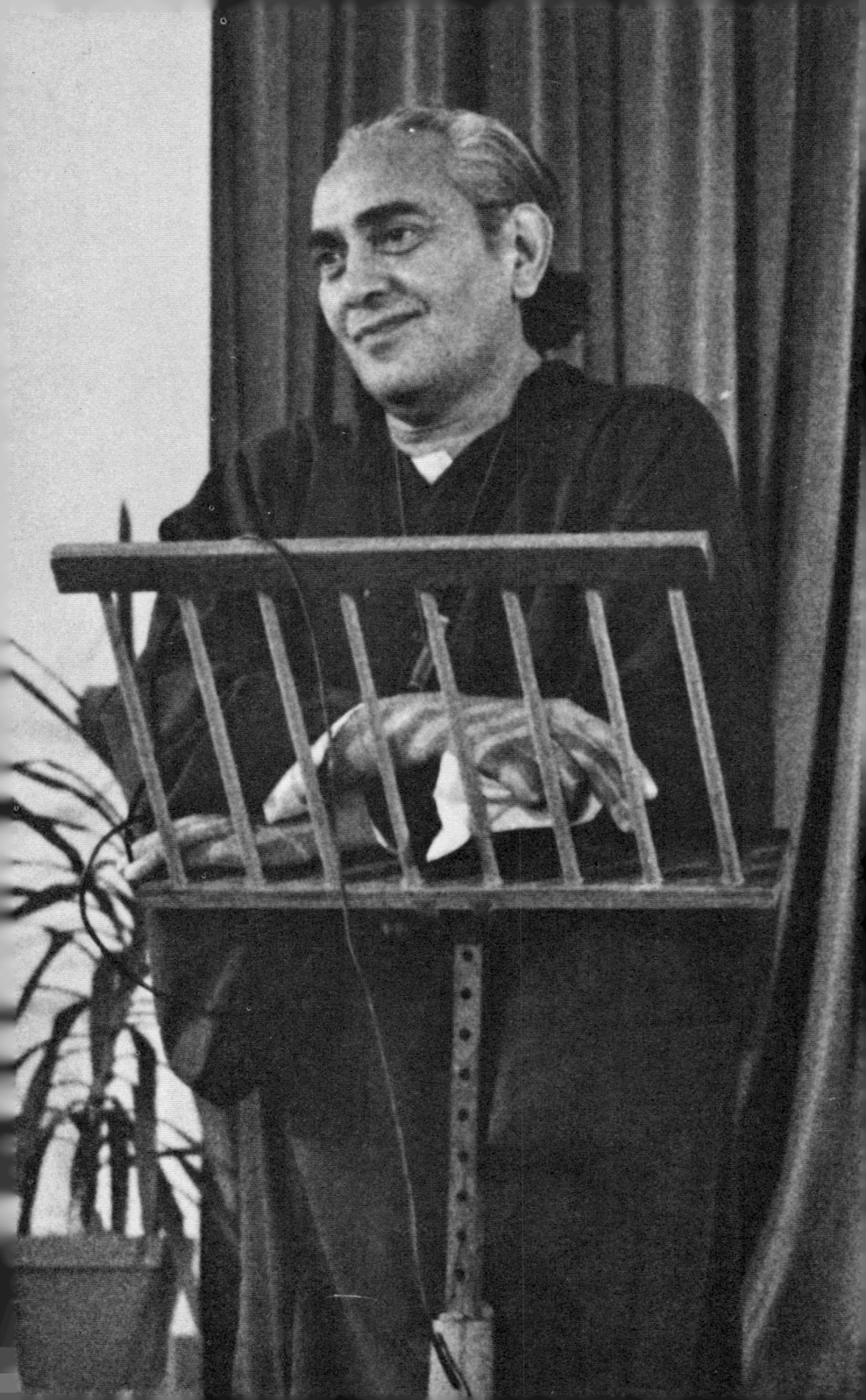

Questions on Spiritual Practice

Published in the Himalayan News, *October, 1977, and January, 1978*

Q: I have heard that you should meditate facing the sun— East in the morning and West in the evening—but that facing North is the best. I feel unsure of the best direction to face for meditation. Can it be changed in the evening and morning, or should it always be the same?

A: While sitting in meditation in the morning and evening, facing East and West, respectively, is considered to be good, but for a true meditator, directions do not mean much. Meditation is a technique that leads one beyond the sense of time, space, and causation, as well as the sense of direction. A comfortable and steady posture should be practiced regularly; it should not be changed again and again. Your seat should be on a firm cushion or folded blanket. Sitting on a hard chair or the floor is not healthy in the long run.

Q: What are the proper items to place on an altar for meditation, and what is their spiritual meaning?

A: You can use an altar for meditation, but it is not necessary. To create a spiritual environment, some students find benefit in meditating before an altar. If you are accustomed to do so, your altar should have flowers and a gentle candle light in a quiet and calm atmosphere.

Q: Is it helpful to have a mantra for meditation, and why? Can one use so ham *or should he have his own mantra?*

A: It is very helpful to have a mantra, for the mantra is a guide, and the mind spontaneously starts meditating on it. It is a necessary means in the journey that helps one to fathom the many subtle levels of consciousness. Breath awareness is important for making the mind one-pointed and inward, and you can coordinate *so ham* with your inhalation and exhalation if you want. Remembering your mantra according to the instructions given to you by your teacher is more helpful than any information you can gain through books. Mantras are effective if you understand the science of mantras. Your teacher should be able to explain to you about your mantra, its usage, and its application.

Q: Can you explain how meditation is not just for Hindus? My family is very orthodox and thinks I have left the church. Are there passages in the Bible and in Jewish literature that refer to meditation as a sanctioned method of worship?

A: Meditation is for all human beings and not for Hindus only. It helps one gain control over the roving habits of the mind. For peace of mind and happiness, meditation is very beneficial. Meditation is not religious, and it does not oppose any religion or church. In the Bible it is said, "Be still and know that I am God" (Psalm 46:10). To sit down in a calm and quiet place, steadily and comfortably, is called stilling the body. To calm down the breath is also necessary. These two preliminary steps help you to still the mind, and then the center of consciousness will reveal itself to you.

Q: Is there such a thing as a healing prayer or a healing touch? What happens? Can anyone do it for anyone else? Is love all that is required? What is the "energy" they speak of as the healing power? How can we become healers, and can we heal ourselves? Are there special ways or should you just try your best and see?

A: All human beings are fully equipped with healing potential, and prayer definitely helps. With the help of prayer, one can heal oneself. If you are very selfless and have compassion for the people whom you want to heal, they definitely will be benefited. Unconditional faith is one of the important qualities you should develop in your heart, and love is the mother of all energy and all healing powers. You are already healing yourselves, and when you become aware of this fact you become a self-healer. There are many methods of healing, but strong faith in God within is the highest of all.

Q: When one is stuck on a "blah plateau" in one's practice and does not seem to be advancing, should he just wait it out, or are there methods he can use to progress further?

A: Sometimes it is natural for students to think that their progress is at a standstill. Patience and sincerity toward one's practice are two essential and preliminary steps. Sometimes desires interfere and distract the mind. One should learn to watch one's actions, speech, thoughts, emotions, and desires; then there will be no obstacles.

Q: A friend with whom I meditate bends forward and then jerks back into place from time to time. Is he falling asleep? Is he sitting incorrectly? Or is his kundalini awakening? Should I touch his elbow and make him aware of this when it happens? It's been going on for a year now.

A: Jerks and bending forward in meditation are signs of not having a steady mind and of not preparing yourself physically. Please encourage him to correct his dietary habits and learn to strengthen his desire for meditation. He will get over this problem. Keeping his head, neck, and trunk straight and sitting in an easy and steady posture are equally important. Falling asleep is because of inertia. Do not be misguided and think that this is a sign or symptom of kundalini awakening. It is possible to awaken kundalini, but steadiness, a one-pointed mind, and a strong desire to tread the systematic path of this science are important.

Q: Is samadhi attained or received? It seems the harder I try to meditate, the more it escapes me. But when I let go and just sit there, I go deeper. What technique is best to show an effort on my part but not be pushy?

A: Samadhi is neither attained nor received. It is the expansion of the individual mind to the realization of the cosmic mind. Do not struggle with your mind, and slowly learn to expand the consciousness. Do not overdo or miss your practices. They are to be done punctually, regularly, with firm faith and love.

Q: Can someone overdo karma yoga, or should some time be given for meditation as well?

A: Karma yoga is a must, and it should be performed selflessly and skillfully. Performing karma yoga selflessly and skillfully is called meditation in action. Sometimes silence makes one aware of one's own duty, and it is also essential.

Q: What should be done about intense feelings of jealousy?

A: Jealousy is a poison one creates for oneself. It is a weakness that creates a barrier on the path of spirituality. Those who are self-centered and selfish are jealous of each others' progress. This is an incompetency that should be removed by positive thinking and realizing one's own weakness. Do not compare yourself with others. Watch your mind, action, and speech.

Q: How many reincarnations must a person go through?

A: For an ignorant individual, reincarnation is the only way. One who is realized, however, obtains freedom from the chain of births and deaths. An enlightened one, if he chooses to come to help others, can reincarnate, but this is his choice.

Q: How can we repay our parents in terms of karma for all the good they have done for us?

A: Serving one's parents is the only way to express one's gratitude and repay our debts. Blessed are those who serve their parents and enjoy doing so.

Q: Why is it harmful to compare ourselves with others, especially in spiritual practice?

A: On the path of spirituality, there can be no such comparison. The path of self-enlightenment starts with self-analysis, then self-control, and finally self-enlightenment. Why do you want to compare yourself with others? Comparing yourself with the sages will positively inspire you, but comparing yourself wth the mundane symbols of the world will mislead you.

Q: How can one build a trust that he is on the right spiritual path? What about fears that seem to hold one back?

A: Fear invites danger. Fear is the most important aspect of ignorance. It means non-trusting of the reality within. Self-reliance and constant awareness will help one in building trust.

Q: As one becomes aware of the negative tendencies in one's thinking, how can these be changed into positive tendencies and cheerfulness?

A: Negative and positive tendencies exist in everyone. Those who practice spirituality and have some aim in life will focus on that aim and direct their resources to fulfilling it. For such a person, negativity becomes meaningless. Positive thinking helps one in all phases of life.

Q: We are used to thinking of God as the Father, but in the East, God is thought of as the Divine Mother. Should we change the deity to whom we pray? Which is better?

A: God is a father, mother, a friend, and is everything. Do not identify yourself with any particular thought pattern, for God is truth alone.

Q: Does a mantra link one with his or her chosen ideal?

A: If a mantra is properly practiced, it becomes a staff of life and directs one at all times.

Second Congress Theme

Second International Congress, Pick-Congress Hotel, Chicago, Illinois, June 16, 1977

In this modern world, our inner and outer conditions and our values have changed dramatically from earlier times. We live in an age that is governed by time. The fast pace in which we live keeps us constantly busy. Modern people have become oriented toward an external way of life, and with this development, the physical and psychological health of human beings is degenerating. But one who is concerned with modern conditions and has studied them in their historical context understands that we are going through a period of transition to achieve something higher—another step of civilization, a civilization in which there is a sense of mutual understanding and good will as well as mental, emotional, and physical well-being.

We have done a great deal of research on matter and energy to bring us many comforts. But this one-sided approach only helps us to expand our consciousness externally. Today we seem to be suffering more internally than externally. Despite all of our progress and external comforts, people are still suffering internally in the same ways they were five thousand years ago. This is because we have not studied our internal states and the methods for their regulation with the same vigor that we have put forward to study and control the external world. More research on all levels of internal processes is essential if we are to make progress in eliminating human suffering.

The Himalayan Institute is concerned with bringing together

scientists and clinicians of different fields and disciplines to work with each other and exchange their knowledge, practical methods, and approaches to holistic health. Our aim is to experiment with, document, and apply the methods of meditational therapy in many situations where humanity suffers. Our Institute is health oriented. It is directed toward helping the people of our society to achieve physical, mental, and spiritual health. We have found that meditation, combined with diet, nutrition, exercise, and breathing techniques, helps one to maintain a productive, healthy, and creative life. Meditation is useful for curing many of the psychosomatic diseases that plague modern humanity. In addition to helping to relieve anxiety, hypertension, headaches, and a variety of psychophysiological disorders, it has also been of significant benefit in the treatment of drug addiction, and it has considerable potential in psychotherapy and biofeedback.

Tranquility and peace of mind are essential for people to be creative and helpful to themselves and others, and meditation is a definite method that brings greater tranquility. It should be included in health programs all over the world. If it were widely taught and practiced, perhaps people would not become so dependent on external means of suppressing suffering but would learn to regulate their internal states to achieve a true sense of well-being.

Meditation helps one to know and acquire control over various levels of mind. It makes one self-reliant and leads one toward a self-training program. It is a spontaneous, automatic process for expanding awareness and understanding all the levels of consciousness. It is like a ladder that takes you from where you are at present and gives you the capacity for attaining higher and higher rungs of real fulfillment.

Meditation is the finest of all therapies. It is a complete and integrated therapy. During this International Congress on Meditation-Related Therapies, you will have a chance to learn about its broad range of application, its close relationship to many forms of therapeutic intervention that are current today, and the way in which meditation can extend these forms of therapy to lead humanity toward its goal of fully realizing its hidden potential.

I would like to welcome all the delegates and participants from various parts of the world. This is an opportunity for all of us to learn, participate in, and enjoy the various approaches that will be discussed here. I hope that you will find this time rewarding and that you will be able to apply what you learn here in your own work and in your daily life. I thank all the speakers and the spiritual leaders for their kind participation in this Congress.

Calm Down Now

Published in the Seventh Congress Souvenir Volume, June, 1982

In the rush and roar of modern civilization, humanity has lost awareness of the gifts it has received from nature. In the cycle of evolution, man has been equipped to know—and to know that he knows—how to use his mind, speech, and action to realize the true meaning of life. But today man has become a victim of modern culture, which is materially oriented, and he has forgotten the aim of his life. He has forgotten that external attainments and material gains are but means and not the end. What good are these means without any aim? Such a person does not know how to relax. For relaxation, one must learn how to release stress and strain on all three levels: muscle, nervous system, and mind. Meditational therapy is the best therapy in the world for releasing stress and strain, and relaxation is the first rung on the ladder of meditation. This positively releases tension.

It has been examined and verified through scientific exploration that more than eighty percent of all diseases are due to stress and strain that originate in the mind and reflect on the body. Meditational therapy is a unique exercise that reduces much stress and disease. It can definitely benefit you, but first you have to learn to work with yourself. If you are dependent on a therapist all the time, that is not true therapy. Without a self-training program, you will never understand your internal states and know yourself on all levels.

Mental health is more important than physical health

243

because physical health is mainly dependent on mental health. It is therefore important to cultivate mental attitudes that insure a steady and tranquil mind before you turn your attention to physical health. The mind and body interact to a greater degree than is normally understood. If the mind is constantly subject to disturbing emotions and thoughts, the resulting bodily disturbances cannot be combated by using physical treatments alone.

Modern people are suffering so much from stress that their entire energy is being channeled for stress management only. They do not have time for self-enlightenment. Everyone wants to be free from stress, but most people have not tried to understand where and how their stress originates. Therefore, they do not know how to be free from that stress, and so they do not make any efforts to be free from it. They are indecisive, and indecisiveness means conflict, which is the source of stress, so more stress is created. People are caught in a snare of problems caused by their actions and thinking. All the various therapy courses are trying to help people release stress, but what about the whole life's course? If one's whole life can be spent in stress management to reduce that strain that we are creating for ourselves all the time, then when will one find time and opportunity to attain the purpose of life? We should take time to think again.

The representatives of the various nations of the world who have impact on the masses should sit down calmly and understand the destiny of humankind. They should ask, "Where are we leading the masses?" So far, there is no nation that can be considered to be totally free from the confusions and miseries created by the way of life its citizens lead. Some nations are better than others in many respects. Some are economically and technologically progressive, and others suffer on account of the lack of external resources. But self-created suffering exists everywhere; human society is still functioning on the gross levels of life. We human beings have not yet been able to create a civilized society that knows the value of a tranquil and balanced life, a society in which all live happily and lovingly, without hatred, jealousy, and turmoil.

We have done much research on three levels—mind, matter, and energy—and we have been successful in exploring some of the components of existence, such as the atom. We have broken the atom, and we have gone on to the nucleus, and now we have started breaking the nucleus. We have been doing all of this through our advanced technology by using our human skills. But we are creating more problems for human growth instead of helping humanity to rise to the level of universal consciousness. We should be searching for the Ultimate Reality, but the scientists and philosophers of the modern world say that there is nothing like an Ultimate Reality. Otherwise, they say, Americans would have found it long ago. They have gone to the moon and sent satellites to several of the planets, but they have not found the Ultimate Reality. We have done enough research on matter, energy, and mind, but we have not done any research on that source which is called intuition. And we have not tapped that infinite source which is called the intuitive library within us. There is no particular school that helps students go to that source.

Sooner or later human destiny is bound to attain a state in which we will all learn to live happily and to understand each other. It will happen when that avenue which is called intuitive power, intuitive knowledge, is opened to us. We know a way to attain that, and it is to calm down the body, senses, and mind with mental effort so that one is allowing the real knowledge that is hidden behind to come forward. This is an inward path. One has to learn to calm down so that one can learn to be active but under control in the external world. Not a single activity should be uncontrolled, because uncontrolled, undirected, and disorderly activity causes stress and strain. One should learn to use that faculty which helps one in discriminating what is helpful from what is not helpful. One must learn how to decide things on time and how to allow one's other faculties to function freely and not to go under the strain of conflicts. In this way, one can attain a state that is free from all pains and miseries.

Pain is a relative term, no matter whether it is physical or mental. Anyone can eliminate his pain if he understands how to do it. One's whole energy is being dissipated by the mind, but there are other avenues of knowledge that can make humankind happy, that lead to a final destination that is the highest, purest state of knowledge. But one cannot attain that through the mind. Many great poets and sages say that their knowledge is not knowledge through the mind. Their knowledge is beyond the mind; it is that knowledge which is free from the relative terms of pain and pleasure. It is beyond the fields of mind. But if one is not controlling the mind, if one's mind is not orderly, if one has not disciplined the mind, then the mind will never allow one to go beyond. It will always stand like a wall between oneself and the Reality.

The human mind creates our worries and problems so that we do not even know how to enjoy the last moments of life. When all the oil of an oil lamp is consumed and the last light shines, it flits. But that doesn't happen with human beings. The last drop of the fuel of life bottled in the body is not consumed properly because one comes here for a certain purpose, and instead of attaining that purpose, one does something different. He becomes attached and forgets his goal. Sense objects, which are considered to be givers of joy and pleasure, thus change the course of human research. Instead of researching the inner levels of life and reaching to the fountain of consciousness, people collect the objects of sense gratification.

A human being actually needs to establish a balance between internal and external life. A great disagreement seems to lie between these two aspects of life. Human society has yet to develop a specific way or program that could be included in the modern educational system. Such a program would prevent millions from having stress and the psychosomatic diseases that have made modern people their victims.

Mantra and Meditation

Published as the Introduction to Mantra and Meditation *by Usharbudh Arya (1981)*

Mantra and Meditation is a book that will dispel the darkness of ignorance of many students who are confused. This book can lead to understanding and knowledge, and an ability to practice the science of meditation. When a meditator probes into the inner levels of his being and explores the unknown dimensions of interior life, he needs a systematic and scientific method that can lead him to the next state of experience. Then he can go beyond all the levels of his unconscious mind and establish himself in his essential nature.

From childhood onward, we are taught to examine and understand things in the external world, but nobody teaches us to look within and understand the mind and its various states. A human being, after examining the objects of the external world, finds that he has not yet understood and known himself or his internal states. Anyone who has examined the objects of the external world and their transitory nature understands that life has more to give, and then he starts searching within himself. In order to do research in the interior world, we have to apply an exact science if we really want to know the center of consciousness hidden deep in the inner recesses of our being. Many students out of curiosity or excitement are turning toward meditative methods and trying to understand them as means of knowing their internal states. Some of these students persist, but others give up exploring their inner dimensions.

In this book, Dr. Arya explains that all the existing spiritual traditions of the world use a syllable, a sound, a word, or set of words called *mantra* as a bridge to cross the mire of delusion and go to the other shore of life. *Mantra setu* is that which helps the meditator make the mind one-pointed and inward, and then finally leads to the center of consciousness, the deep recesses of eternal silence where peace, happiness, and bliss reside.

Many spiritual traditions have somehow, somewhere already lost this science of mantra. They remain scratching the surface in the external world, just muttering a few certain words in their own language, which they call a prayer. Prayer definitely purifies the way of the soul, but the method of meditation is a systematized way of exploring the interior self and inner states of human life. There is a vast difference between prayer and meditation. Prayer is a petition to someone with a particular desire to be fulfilled, while the method of meditation leads one from the gross self to the subtlemost Self. Those who are students of life can clearly understand the difference between prayer and meditation. Prayer, meditation, and contemplation are different tools, different ways for attaining the goal of life.

It is clear that the method of meditation is not any ritual belonging to any particular religion, culture, or group. Our tradition is a meditative tradition that does not oppose any religion or culture, but teaches one to systematically explore the inner dimensions. Many Westerners are scared of the word *meditation* and say that it is from an Eastern tradition, forgetting that the Bible clearly says, "Be still and know that I am God." How to be still is the method of meditation. Even imitating the way others are meditating is very relaxing. Meditation is beneficial for physical, mental, and spiritual health.

The Method of Meditation

In meditation, one has to learn to be still first. This begins with a physical stillness. First, the student is guided by a competent teacher to keep the head, neck, and trunk straight. According to the tradition that we follow, the *asana* or meditative posture is carefully selected according to the nature and capacity of the student. It is not changed; one posture alone is practiced until one becomes accomplished at it. After accomplishing stillness with the help of the meditative posture, the student understands the obstacles arising from muscle twitching, tremors occurring in various parts of the body, shaking, and itching.

These obstacles arise from lack of discipline because the body has never been trained to be placed in a still position. We are trained to move in the external world faster and faster, but nobody trains us how to be still. For being still, an orderly habit should be formed, and for forming this habit, one should learn to be regular and punctual in practicing the same posture at the same time and at the same place until the body habits stop rebelling against the discipline being given to it. This primary step, though very basic, is very important. It should not be ignored. Otherwise the student will not be able to reap the desired fruits, and his or her efforts will be wasted.

We should learn about mantra and meditation by studying only those books that have been written by meditators, and we should avoid the trash literature written for commercial use. A book definitely guides and inspires the student, but finally, the book of life seems to be the most important. The highest of all books is the book of life. Meditators and contemplators alone can unfold the pages of this book.

Contemplation and meditation are two different words and methods. Meditation is a definite method like a ladder with many rungs that finally leads to the roof from where one can see the vast horizon above and below, here, there, and everywhere. Contemplation also uses a systematic method; it examines the principles of life and the universe, constantly assimilating these ideas and transforming the whole personality. Those who are fully dedicated and have given their whole life for Self-realization use both methods—meditation in deep silence and contemplation in daily life. Contemplation is seeking and searching for truth, and meditation is practicing and experiencing truth. The Lord of life is truth. Let us practice truth with mind, action, and speech.

Secondly, love is the Light of Lights. Let us radiate this love by not hurting, harming, injuring, and killing others. Such ideas, if practiced in daily life, are called contemplation.

We believe that all great religions have come from one and the same Reality. We also believe that without knowing the Absolute Truth, the purpose of life cannot be accomplished. Though the schools of meditation and contemplation are two different schools, they can both help students go beyond and establish themselves in their essential nature, which is peace, happiness, and bliss. It is the mind that stands as a wall between apparent reality and Absolute Reality. Mantra is a means, meditation is a method, and the constant state of awareness of Absolute Truth is the attainment that fulfills the purpose of life.

This method of meditation is an inner method that has been thoroughly explored for centuries together by the great sages. There are various channels of knowledge—knowledge through the mind, knowledge through the senses, knowledge through instinct—but the finest of all is the intuitive knowledge that has been the guide of all great people in the past. To reach this infinite library within is not so easy; it is a difficult task, but it is not impossible. Just as a scholar works hard to accomplish a task in any academic field, the meditator should also collect the data from various traditions and examine the methods before applying a particular suitable method. So often, students talk only of this method and that method, and they get confused by the sayings and writings of modern writers and speakers.

Meditative scholars instruct the student in how to be free from external influences and how to follow the primary steps so that body, senses, and mind are prepared for meditative experiences. If these preliminaries are ignored, then the student might waste years and years in hallucination and fantasy just to feed the ego and not have any valid experiences. A valid experience is an experience that guides the student. Human beings have experiences on many levels, but all experiences do not guide them. A valid experience is so clear that one does not need any external evidence to support that experience. Such an experience is gained only when the student attains a state of equanimity and tranquillity.

As a student makes sincere efforts to find a right teacher and a suitable method of meditation, so actually a teacher also remains in search of a good student who is fully prepared to take this voyage—the voyage from the known to the unknown. Doubts and fears may arise on various occasions, but when students decide to tread the path of meditation, they honestly prepare and discipline themselves. They examine all their instrumentation in the laboratory of life. Body, senses, breath, and mind are attuned toward meditation only. Those who have been researchers and have examined the external joys find that the highest of all joys is meditation, and this joy leads to that eternal joy called *samadhi*. Such great ones like to keep their eyes partially closed, peeping into the innermost light that shines within this frame of life.

According to our tradition, which is purely a meditative tradition more than five thousand years old, mantra and meditation are inseparable just like two sides of a coin. Some of the shallow methods that have been taught lead one only so far, but the systematic method that is explained in this book can help a student to attain the highest of all states. For practicing the method of meditation, one should not dive into shallow waters, for the pearls of life are found in the deep ocean of life and not in the ponds, lakes, and rivers.

The Inner Sounds

During deep meditation, the great sages heard certain sounds, called mantras. In the Bible, it is said that those who have an ear to hear will hear. When the mind becomes attuned, it becomes capable of hearing the voice of the unknown. The sounds that are heard in such a state do not belong to any particular language, religion, or tradition.

There are two types of sounds. The sounds that are created by the external world and heard by the ears are different than the sounds heard in deep meditation. Such inner sounds are called *anahata nada*—the sound of drums without drums. The inner sounds heard by the sages in deep meditation do not vibrate exactly like sound vibrates in the external world. These inner sounds have a leading quality; they lead the meditator toward the center of silence within. The following simile can help you to understand this. Imagine that you are standing on the bank of a river and you hear the current as it flows. If you follow the river upstream, you will come to its origin. There you will find that there is no sound. In the same way, a mantra leads the mind to the silence within. That state is called "soundless sound."

The mantra imparted by a teacher to a student is not at all a commercial proposition. It is more like a prescription given to a patient. There are innumerable sounds, each with different effects. The teacher must find out which best suits a particular student according to his or her attitudes, emotions, desires, and habits.

A mantra has four bodies, or *koshas* (sheaths). First, as a word, it has a meaning; another more subtle form is its feeling; still more subtle is a deep, intense, and constant awareness or presence; and the fourth or most subtle level of the mantra is soundless sound. Many students continue repeating or muttering their mantra throughout life, but they never attain a state of *ajapa japa*—that state of constant awareness without any effort. Such a student strengthens his awareness but meditates on the gross level only.

The mantras used for meditation in silence are special sets of sounds that do not obstruct and disturb the flow of breath but rather help regulate the breath and lead to *sushumna* awakening, where breath flows from both nostrils equally. This is a state in which the breath and mind function in complete harmony. Application of sushumna is a joyous state of mind. After attaining this state, the mind is voluntarily disconnected from the dissipation of the senses. Then the student has to deal with the thoughts coming forward from the storehouse of merits and demerits—the unconscious mind. This is a vast reservoir where we store the impressions of our lifetime. The conscious mind is in the habit of recalling these memories from the deep levels of the unconscious. Mantra helps one to go beyond this process. Mantra creates a new groove, and the mind begins to spontaneously flow into the groove it creates. When the mind becomes concentrated, one-pointed, and inward, it peers into the latent part of the unconscious, and there it sooner or later finds a glittering light.

The most important role that mantra plays is during the transition period that every human being has to go through: death. A dying person wants to communicate with his loved ones. The attachments that we create for mortal things and people produce serious and painful troubles for a dying person. For lack of practice of meditation and self-experience, for lack of a philosophy, which ought to have been built during one's lifetime, attachments become very painful. Death itself is not painful, but the fear of death is very painful, especially for those who have not pondered over the mystery of birth, death, and the hereafter. In such cases, these last moments of life cause extreme discomfort and even affect the voyage after death. This subtle observation leads me to declare that the depth of prayer, contemplation, and meditation should be taught, practiced, and experienced with full honesty, clarity of mind, and one-pointedness. A dying man's senses do not function properly. He gradually loses his eyesight, his tongue mumbles words that are not understood by others, and he is unable to express his thoughts through speech and actions. This painful and pitiable situation scares the mind in the case of non-meditators. But, if someone remembers the mantra for a long time in such a state of loneliness, the mantra starts leading him, and this miserable period of loneliness and agony is over.

One single thought pattern is strengthened by remembering the mantra; it becomes predominant and leads the individual sufferer to the abode of peace, happiness, and bliss. This experience has been validated by me personally after witnessing the death of many sages. I have also witnessed the death of many rich men, scientists, and so-called academicians, and I found them going through miserable agonies. Their facial expressions and helplessness were quite a proof to me that they did not prepare themselves for this last moment of life. I am not recommending any particular mantra coming from any particular source or tradition, but the magnanimity of mantra and meditation can be examined if you quietly observe a sage, a rich man, and an intellectual when they are on their death beds.

The Lineage of Meditation

Christians, Jews, Buddhists, and Sufis all have their traditions, but a systematic meditation system has been lost in those great cultures. I don't accept meditation as a part of any particular culture or religion, but I view it as a scientific method and a prime necessity for everyone all over the world.

According to our lineage, there are two branches of teachers. One teaches the scriptures, observing austerities, and following the path of renunciation. The other branch is a branch of meditators and contemplators doing documentation experiments and scientifically collecting data on all levels of life—physical, energy level, level of sense perception, the way things are perceived on the mental level, and finally on a spiritual level.

This book is a gift from our unbroken lineage of meditators to its readers, to the students who are treading the inner path of light. For doing inner research, mantra and meditation are the greatest aids to the seekers. Let you not disturb your religion. But let you learn to know yourself on all levels. Let you also be aware of those fanatics who tell you not to meditate, for meditation is a condensed, deep, and intense form of prayer that is not a person-centered prayer but is a God-centered prayer.

One who lives in the world can attain the highest state of samadhi through meditation. He is here, yet there; he lives in the world, yet above. He includes all and excludes none. Will there ever be a day when every man, woman, and child begins practicing meditation? As a result, we can all attain the next step of civilization and realize the unity in life. Liberation can be attained here and now.

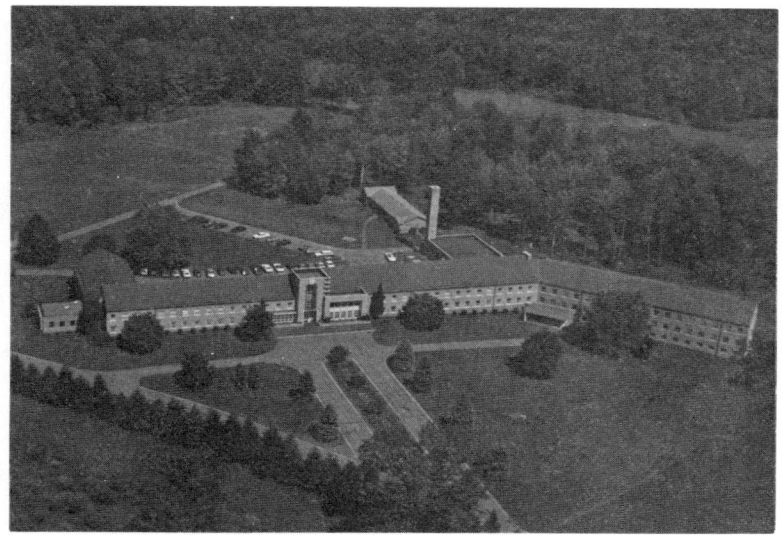

The main building of the national headquarters, Honesdale, Pa.

The Himalayan Institute

The Himalayan International Institute of Yoga Science and Philosophy of the U.S.A. is a nonprofit organization devoted to the scientific and spiritual progress of modern humanity. Founded in 1971 by Sri Swami Rama, the Institute combines Western and Eastern teachings and techniques to develop educational, therapeutic, and research programs for serving people in today's world. The goals of the Institute are to teach meditational techniques for the growth of individuals and their society, to make known the harmonious view of world religions and philosophies, and to undertake scientific research for the benefit of humankind.

This challenging task is met by people of all ages, all walks of life, and all faiths who attend and participate in the Institute courses and seminars. These programs, which are given on a continuing basis, are designed in order that one may discover for oneself how to live more creatively. In the words of Swami Rama, "By being aware of one's own potential and abilities, one can become a perfect citizen, help the nation, and serve humanity."

The Institute has branch centers and affiliates throughout the United States. The 422-acre campus of the national headquarters, located in the Pocono Mountains of northeastern Pennsylvania, serves as the coordination center for all the Institute activities, which include a wide variety of innovative programs in education, research, and therapy, combining Eastern and Western approaches to self-awareness and self-directed change.

SEMINARS, LECTURES, WORKSHOPS, and CLASSES are available throughout the year, providing intensive training and experience in such topics as Superconscious Meditation, hatha yoga, philosophy, psychology, and various aspects of personal growth and holistic health. The *Himalayan News*, a free bimonthly publication, announces the current programs.

The RESIDENTIAL and SELF-TRANSFORMATION PROGRAMS provide training in the basic yoga disciplines—diet, ethical behavior, hatha yoga, and meditation. Students are also given guidance in a philosophy of living in a community environment.

The PROGRAM IN EASTERN STUDIES AND COM-PARATIVE PSYCHOLOGY is the first curriculum offered by an educational institution that provides a systematic synthesis of Western empirical sciences with Eastern introspective sciences using both practical and traditional approaches to education. The University of Scranton, by an agreement of affiliation with the Himalayan Institute, is prepared to grant credits for coursework in this program, and upon successful completion of the program awards a Master of Science degree.

The five-day STRESS MANAGEMENT/PHYSICAL FIT-NESS PROGRAM offers practical and individualized training that can be used to control the stress response. This includes biofeedback, relaxation skills, exercise, diet, breathing techniques, and meditation.

A yearly INTERNATIONAL CONGRESS, sponsored by the Institute, is devoted to the scientific and spiritual progress of modern humanity. Through lectures, workshops, seminars, and practical demonstrations, it provides a forum for professionals and lay people to share their knowledge and research.

The ELEANOR N. DANA RESEARCH LABORATORY is the psychophysiological laboratory of the Institute, specializing in research on breathing, meditation, holistic therapies, and stress and relaxed states. The laboratory is fully equipped for exercise stress testing and psychophysiological measurements, including brain waves, patterns of respiration, heart rate changes, and muscle tension. The staff investigates Eastern teachings through studies based on Western experimental techniques.

Himalayan Institute Publications

Living with the Himalayan Masters	Swami Rama
Lectures on Yoga	Swami Rama
A Practical Guide to Holistic Health	Swami Rama
Choosing a Path	Swami Rama
Inspired Thoughts of Swami Rama	Swami Rama
Freedom from the Bondage of Karma	Swami Rama
Book of Wisdom (Ishopanishad)	Swami Rama
Enlightenment Without God	Swami Rama
Life Here and Hereafter	Swami Rama
Marriage, Parenthood, and Enlightenment	Swami Rama
Emotion to Enlightenment	Swami Rama, Swami Ajaya
Science of Breath	Swami Rama, Rudolph Ballentine, M.D., Alan Hymes, M.D.
Yoga and Psychotherapy	Swami Rama, Rudolph Ballentine, M.D., Swami Ajaya
Superconscious Meditation	Usharbudh Arya, D.Litt.
Mantra and Meditation	Usharbudh Arya, D.Litt.
Philosophy of Hatha Yoga	Usharbudh Arya, D.Litt.
Meditation and the Art of Dying	Usharbudh Arya, D.Litt.
God	Usharbudh Arya, D.Litt.
Yoga Psychology	Swami Ajaya, Ph.D.
Foundations of Eastern and Western Psychology	Swami Ajaya (ed.)
Psychology East and West	Swami Ajaya (ed.)
Meditational Therapy	Swami Ajaya (ed.)
Diet and Nutrition	Rudolph Ballentine, M.D.
Joints and Glands Exercises	Rudolph Ballentine, M.D. (ed.)
Theory and Practice of Meditation	Rudolph Ballentine, M.D. (ed.)
Freedom from Stress	Phil Nuernberger, Ph.D.
Science Studies Yoga	James Funderburk, Ph.D.
Homeopathic Remedies	Drs. Anderson, Buegel, Chernin
Hatha Yoga Manual I	Samskrti and Veda
Hatha Yoga Manual II	Samskrti and Judith Franks
Seven Systems of Indian Philosophy	R. Tigunait, Ph.D.
Swami Rama of the Himalayas	L. K. Misra, Ph.D. (ed.)
Philosophy of Death and Dying	M. V. Kamath
Practical Vedanta of Swami Rama Tirtha	Brandt Dayton (ed.)
The Swami and Sam	Brandt Dayton
Psychology of the Beatitudes	Arpita, Ph.D.
Himalayan Mountain Cookery	Martha Ballentine
The Yoga Way Cookbook	Himalayan Institute
Inner Paths	Himalayan Institute